International Security, Conflict and Gender

I0039446

This book challenges the conventional security-based international policy frameworks that have developed for dealing with HIV/AIDS during and after conflicts, and examines first-hand evidence and experiences of conflict and HIV/AIDS.

Since the turn of the century, the international policy agenda on security has focused on HIV/AIDS only as a concern for national and international security, ignoring people's particular experiences, vulnerabilities and needs in conflict and post-conflict contexts. Developing a gender-based framework for HIV/AIDS-conflict analysis, this book draws on research conducted in Burundi to understand the implications of post-conflict demobilization and reintegration policies on women and men, and their vulnerability to HIV/AIDS. By centering the argument on personal reflections, this work provides a critical alternative method to engage with conflict and HIV/AIDS, and a much richer understanding of the relationship between the two.

International Security, Conflict and Gender will be of interest to students and scholars of healthcare politics, security and governance.

Hakan Seckinelgin is Senior Lecturer in International Social Policy at the Department of Social Policy, London School of Economics, UK.

Routledge Research in Comparative Politics

International Security, Conflict and Gender

'HIV/AIDS is another war'

Hakan Seckinelgin

Routledge
Taylor & Francis Group

LONDON AND NEW YORK

First published 2012
by Routledge
2 Park Square, Milton Park, Abingdon, Oxfordshire OX14 4RN

Simultaneously published in the USA and Canada
by Routledge
711 Third Avenue, New York, NY 10017

First issued in paperback 2014

Routledge is an imprint of the Taylor & Francis Group, an informa business

British Library Cataloguing in Publication Data
A catalogue record for this book is available from the British Library

Library of Congress Cataloging in Publication Data
Seckinelgin, Hakan, 1969-
    International security, conflict, and gender : "HIV/AIDS is another war" /
Hakan Seckinelgin. – 1st ed.
    p. cm. – (Routledge research in comparative politics ; 50)
    Includes bibliographical references and index.
    1. Conflict management–Great Lakes Region (Africa) 2. Women and
war–Great Lakes Region (Africa) 3. HIV infections–Social aspects–Great
Lakes Region (Africa) 4. AIDS (Disease)–Great Lakes Region (Africa) 5.
Africa–Politics and government–21st century. I. Title.
    HM1126.S43 2012
    362.196'97920096761–dc23
                            2011050781

ISBN: 978-0-415-61570-9 (hbk)
ISBN: 978-1-138-82164-4 (pbk)

Typeset in Times New Roman by
Taylor & Francis Books

In memoriam
Zehra Günemek (1914–96)
Anne-Marie Henry (1924–2011)

Contents

Acknowledgments

This book is based on research conducted in Burundi on conflict, gender and HIV/AIDS. The research was part of *the* AIDS, Security and Conflict Initiative (ASCI) of the Social Science Research Council and 'Clingendael' Netherlands Institute for International Relations for funding this research. In particular, I would like to thank Alex de Waal, Jennifer Klot, Georg Frerks, and Steven Schoofs for their support and enthusiasm for the research. The ASCI report from Burundi contributed to the final report of the program. This report was submitted to UNAIDS and informed the drafting of the United Nations Security Council Resolution 1983 on HIV/AIDS in June 2011. The research produced much more than what was in the Burundi report. Burundians were very generous with their time to talk, in many cases, about very difficult experiences of conflict and HIV/AIDS. The book was written to bring out as much as possible from their in-depth reflections, to challenge the broader debates on conflict and HIV/AIDS. The book follows their reflections to draw out the major challenges these pose for international policy thinking.

I am deeply grateful to all those who shared their experiences and their hopes with us. In all cases, they wanted to be heard. It was clear that they considered this engagement with us a way of expressing themselves. They did not expect anything in return from their engagements other than being assured that we will let their views be heard. Therefore, this book is written with this understanding, that their voices be heard. Although their names remain anonymous throughout the book I am very grateful to each individual for their time and willingness to engage with this research. The research was a humbling experience.

The research would have been impossible, even if people were willing to talk, without the central contribution of Joseph Bigirumwami and Jill Morris. Both have an openness and passion to engage with people. Both showed great care and sensitivity to people and their conditions. They acted as field researchers conducting the interviews either together or with me as a group. It was a great experience to be in the field with them. Joseph's language skills were indispensable. Jill has a great ability to engage with people on their own terms without being an 'ex-pat'. I am also fortunate to have them as friends. I hope that they find the book true to our aims in the research. I would also like to thank Leanne Bayer, Prudence Marango, Elizabeth McClintock, Kassie McIlvaine, Jean Ndayisenga, Leon Ndikumana, Jean Baptiste Nimubona, Dieudonné Ntamahangarizo, Dieudonné Ntanago, Jean Bosco Nzigamasabo, and Aline Rivuzimana for their ongoing support throughout the research. I am also grateful to Leanne and Liz who were our *surrogate family*, which everyone needs, in the field.

Back at the LSE, I would like to thank the generations of students in the Department of Social Policy, taking Social Policy and Development and Social Policy Research degrees, who heard me talk about this research, Burundians and their experiences. Some of the ideas that inform my analysis here were presented to them and I thank them for their questions and engagement with my discussions. I would also like to thank Nancy Cartwright for her invitation to give lectures and seminars in the LSE's Department of Philosophy, Logic and Scientific Method on how in this research people's experiences challenge the way evidence and policy are generally considered in the field. I am also grateful to her for the ongoing discussions we have on these issues, they are an important source of my thinking and motivation. I would also like to thank my colleagues Dianne Josephs, David Lewis, Eileen Munro and Wendy Sigle-Rushton for their general support throughout this research and writing process. I am also grateful to my mother, Beyhan Seckinelgin, for her constant support.

In the last few years I have also presented parts of the discussion in various conferences and seminars: the International Studies Association in 2009, I want to thank all the participants on the panel *Women, peace, and Security: Issues in Post- and Non-conflict Situations*; in the Anthro-Politics Workshop 2009 in Roskilde University, Denmark, I am grateful to Christian Lund and Lisa Ann Richey for the invitation and participants for their comments; in ESRC/BISA seminar on African Agency: Transnational Security Challenges in June 2011 in the University of Kent, Canterbury I would like to thank Anne Hammerstad and Sophie Harman for the invitation and also all the participants for their useful comments.

I would like to thank also my editors at Routledge, Heidi Bagtazo, Alexander Quayle, Hannah Shakespeare, Paola Celli and Ann Grant, for their enthusiasm about this project and for their support all through the process. Thanks are also due to three anonymous reviewers who considered the book proposal and the sample chapters. They provided interesting questions and comments which made the analysis stronger.

Damien Fennell talked, discussed, argued and listened to many of the life stories and the thoughts they sparked since before the inception of this research wherever we travelled, walked and in our daily life. He read all the chapters at least once and his comments and suggestions for ideas and clarity of expressions were most valuable. His support and companionship nurture my work and life. Of course, as always, the responsibility for all the shortcomings of the book remains mine.

The book is dedicated to two grandmothers: Zehra Günemek (1914–96), my grandmother, *Anneannem,* and Anne-Marie Henry (1924–2011), Damien's grandmother, *Mamie.* They never met each other, lived in different countries, but they were inspiring people in similar ways. They were two very strong women who engaged with the fast changing reality of their world with great enthusiasm to the last. While engaging with the norms of their society they were also changing the ways in which those norms were used for their and their families benefit. I always had very interesting discussions with *Anneannem* on issues that I now realize to be about gender and power. *Mamie* was the same, she was a keen follower of politics and loved books. I began writing parts of this book while away on a break with *Mamie* in Maderia and unfortunately completed it in Paris at the time of her unexpected passing in the middle of November 2011. They both loved the sun.

November 2011 London

An earlier version of Chapter 6 was published as 'What is the evidence that there is no evidence? The link between conflict and HIV/AIDS' in *European Journal of Development Research*, 2010, 22 (3): 363–81.

Introduction

In early April 2007 on a return journey from a research trip to Rwanda and Kenya I was staying with a friend in Bujumbura, Burundi, as I had done in the previous couple of years. My friend was the head of an international contractor which was working to deliver a part of the post-conflict disarmament, demobilization, and reintegration (DDR)-related social package to the ex-combatants in a number of regions in Burundi. This included the region called *Bujumbura-Rural* immediately in the area surrounding the capital, *Bujumbura Marie* (Bujumbura). On this visit we agreed to travel out of Bujumbura since the security situation had improved compared with travel in previous years. Their offices were in central Bujumbura not too far from the main market in a modern office building which they were sharing with a number of other international organizations. The building was surrounded by a high perimeter wall on one side and the other side backed on to the gardens of residential houses. On this particular warm afternoon we were sitting in my friend's office with another colleague who was working for an international non-governmental organization (NGO) on a fact-finding mission in Burundi at the time, chatting about our impending trip, their work, and the challenges they face. Suddenly we were aware of shouts and very loud arguing from the front of the building. As there were guards controlling access to the front yard of the building we were wondering what might be happening out there. My friend thought that it might have been a repeat of the events of the previous week when a large number of frustrated ex-combatants who had been waiting to receive their reinsertion packages protested in front of their offices and attempted to storm the building by climbing over the perimeter wall. The police had been called to control the crowd and my friend had had a discussion with them over the wall. She pointed out to them that their work was dependent on the government releasing funds and that was where the delay had occurred. The situation was diffused. While we were discussing this, another colleague came in to the office to tell us that this was a smaller group and that they were insisting on seeing the head of the mission and were otherwise refusing to leave the compound. My friend agreed to meet them.

We stood back near to my friend's desk while six ex-combatants entered the office with three others working for an international contractor. My friend and her second in command, her *chief de cabinet* who was Burundian and translated the discussion, were seated at the top of the table. We were standing just behind them and the ex-combatants were seated around the table. One of them began to speak. He was clearly articulate and was considered their spokesperson. He pointed out that nobody cared about them, they fought and now people were just trying to ignore them. He said that they needed money but they also needed people to listen to them. He carried on talking about the problems they faced on a daily basis to survive. It was a very calm and rather reflective process. I found this very interesting. They had come to demand their reinsertion package but then mostly talked about things bothering them in general. I realized that both my friend and her colleague were acting as counselors to this group of ex-combatants. It was during this conversation I found myself thinking for the first time about the gap between these people's needs, as related to the way they considered their wellbeing, and how international security concerns were engaging with these people and their needs under the category of ex-combatants. The experience we had that afternoon was repeated a number of times over the following days as we travelled to Makamba via Nynza Lac to meet with various ex-combatant groups and deliver their insertion package installments that were given to them, in kind, to develop small businesses.

In Nyanza Lac, a group of ex-combatants were awaiting us for a meeting, and a similar discussion took place in the restaurant chosen as the place of the meeting. In a small hillside village outside Nynza Lac we were delivering paraffin as an in-kind insertion installment to an ex-combatant who had developed a candle-making workshop in a small shed by the village square. While we were waiting outside the village for someone to give us directions to the hillside to meet the ex-combatant, people came around to talk. One of them was a young man of 17 years and he wanted to talk in English. He wanted to find a way of working in the town and to save money to buy a motorcycle to carry goods. He was asking for ideas. Then we drove to the hillside. As we got out of our cars onlookers wondered what we were delivering, and children ran down the hill to meet us. The person we went to see was talking to one of the workers in Kirundi. However, when my friend addressed him in English he reacted but still insisted in speaking in Kirundi. This was interesting. When she asked him whether he spoke English and whether he was a returnee he did not want to talk about it. This suggested that he was indeed able to speak English and had learned to do so in Tanzania. He was clearly a returnee who did not want this to be obvious to everyone in the village. The complex relationship this man had with his village and the government providing him with his reinsertion package presented me with a challenging view about his livelihood needs. While some of these were material, others were much more social and cultural, underwriting his acceptance on the hillside. Throughout the journey we met many ex-combatants.

Another thing which was very noticeable was the absence of women from these meetings. When we asked, we were told that very few female ex-combatants were formally demobilized and therefore entitled to reinsertion provision. Furthermore, the question of entitlement to these resources by an ex-combatant's wife when he was unwell was also highlighted as an important problem. It transpired that at times the husband's family was trying to capture these resources independent of the needs of his wife and children.

It was very difficult not to have questions about the complexity of people's everyday needs and the implications of the conflict in Burundi. In all of these instances the striking issue was the way people's needs were met materially but little space was available for much more social and psychological needs that had been created by the conflict. Many were happy to be given their insertion packages but also wanted to talk about their experiences both from the period of the conflict and after they had been demobilized. In particular, from the aggressive group we had met at the office in Bujumbura it was very clear that money was part of the issue but also they wanted to be heard and feel part of the community. No doubt they wanted to move beyond the past and get on with their lives. But part of this for many also involved being heard. These encounters were challenging and thought provoking. As a researcher focusing on HIV/AIDS they were making me think about the way they were experiencing the disease and how their feelings and being marginalized might have been making them vulnerable to HIV risks. What was the situation of the women who were so absent from the resource relations initiated by the reinsertion packages? In response to these questions, I was told that many received the HIV/AIDS sensitization program while in the demobilization camps before they were released. The follow-up process around reinsertion did not focus on HIV/AIDS issue. The trip also forced me to think about the debates on international security and HIV/AIDS. Prior to this I had intentionally kept out of this debate, which had gained momentum from about the end of 1990s onwards, and particularly after United Nations Security Council resolution 1308 in 2000 on security and HIV/AIDS. One reason for distancing myself from the debate was the difficulty I had in understanding why analysts wanted to analyze people with HIV and HIV/AIDS as a function of security concerns that were framed according to some state and/or international interests. In my research experience, people's everyday lives and the problems of HIV/AIDS in those lives were somewhat distant from the politics of security as framed in the international fora. The trip and the encounters it provided were profoundly challenging as people's needs revealed significant challenges to international concerns about security and the way they framed dealing with insecurity in Burundi. With these thoughts I returned to London to teach and complete the work that was generated by my research trip before visiting Burundi again.

Unexpectedly, a month later I was asked whether I would consider preparing a research proposal to look at gendered HIV risks in post-conflict Burundi. This was within the AIDS, Security and Conflict Initiative (ASCI). Because of the above-mentioned intentional disengagement from the security debate my response would have been negative to this request if not for the recent encounters in Burundi. This request created an interesting opportunity to engage with the questions that were still in my mind about ex-combatants, HIV and Burundi. With some nervousness that I was getting involved with a study area, Security and HIV/AIDS, which has become a substantive field of analysis in global health, I went ahead with the research. This book is the outcome of this research.

The research and the book

The parameters of the research in Burundi were determined by the context of ASCI, launched by the Social Science Research Council in partnership with the Netherlands Institute for International Relations (Clingendael). The aim of the initiative was to identify and address critical gaps in knowledge in the analysis of the link between HIV/AIDS, security and conflict. It covered four areas: HIV/AIDS in uniformed services; HIV/AIDS, humanitarian crises and post-conflict transitions; HIV/AIDS and fragile states; and gender and cross-cutting issues. The final report was published in 2009 (de Waal *et al.* 2009). The research I proposed was to investigate the post-conflict transition in Burundi with particular emphasis on the relationship between ex-combatants, their re-integration within communities, the changing nature of HIV/AIDS and gender relationships in the country. Specifically the research was focused around three questions:

1 How have HIV/AIDS risks changed with the policies developed in post-conflict Burundi?
2 What are the gender implications of these changes?
3 Are the policies developed in the post-conflict period addressing the necessary structures that have exacerbated HIV/AIDS?

The research was to be based on interviews and discussion groups with different groups of people that included ex-combatants, women who were exposed to the conflict in diverse context, such as rebel camps and in their own communities or in internally displaced people camps, and policy makers. This required a research team able to engage with these groups in their chosen language; this could have been in Kirundi, French or English. I managed to secure two experts as research officers to help with the interviews. The participation of both Joseph Bigirumwami and Jill Morris was critical for the interviews. Joseph is a trained linguist who is a well-known and respected professor of local languages at the University of Burundi. Since the end of the conflict he had worked in the DDR process as an expert respected by many across the conflict divide. Jill had worked as an international NGO officer in Burundi for number of years and was finishing her MSc at the London School of Economics at the time. She knew the context well, and her knowledge was impressively grounded in everyday Burundian social realities and life. Our assumption was that the HIV/AIDS risk had been altered during the conflict, as it had initiated larger socio-political changes that were impacting on gender relations in Burundi.

From the beginning of the research we were aware of the fact that the questions we were interested in could not be tackled by asking them directly because of the perceived sensitivity to HIV/AIDS, gender and conflict in Burundi. Many organizational actors and individuals would not answer or engage with them. There are a number of reasons for this: (a) conflict remains a sensitive issue; (b) HIV/AIDS is a topic difficult to speak openly about; (c) the tendency to talk about 'we' as a collective and difficulty to engage with more individualized questions; (d) the tendency among people to respond to structured questions by giving a response that they feel the researcher is looking for; (e) questions about HIV/AIDS and policies dealing with it in the post-conflict context present a challenge for the political authorities at present; and (f) the political environment in Burundi remains volatile, and civil servants, in particular, are very cautious in answering questions for fear of reprisal. In addition to these complications, another important reason for people's hesitation to engage was similar to an issue highlighted by Barbara Teboh in her research in Cameroon. She states that after approaching people for interviews she was told that people associated 'to interview' with 'to interrogate' (Achebe and Teboh 2007: 68) and did not trust the researcher enough to talk about their experiences. We discussed these constraints at length, thought about the issues we were interested in and how we could ask our various questions of the different groups of people we were going to meet across the country. We decided that the best approach, particularly for people who were not in formal governance structures at that time, was to ask open-ended questions to allow interviewees to talk about their experiences in a life story narrative style. We decided to begin with general questions that were seen as not threatening to individuals and gradually move to more sensitive questions. As a result of this approach, interviews typically took anything between an hour to three hours and, on a few occasions, even longer. In the end we had more people who wanted to talk to us than we anticipated.

It was during the initial interviews and in group meetings that we realized one of our assumptions concerning people's unwillingness to talk about these issues was inaccurate. The reasoning that informed our assumption was that the Burundians were reticent to talk about themselves, particularly in groups, and reticent to talk about gender and HIV. This was not just our assumption: many Burundians and people who have worked in Burundi for a long time insisted that the research was going to be difficult as people do not like talking openly about sensitive issues. We immediately realized at the first group interview that people were keen to talk, and in fact they wanted to talk about their particular experiences. This does not however imply that conversations were in any way easy. Given that we decided to ask people to talk about their experiences, most of the interviews were long and very emotional for all involved. Furthermore, some of the individual and group discussions were emotional since they were difficult to finalize as people wanted to continue talking more.

This process of interviews resulted in us gathering large amounts of information about people's experiences of the conflict in their everyday lives. A resulting challenge was how to report what we had heard. Obioma Nnaemeka talked about how African women's voices were lost in the process of gathering, articulation and dissemination of knowledge (1998: 354). Furthermore, it was clear to us during the research that this silencing also applied to men who were not in power positions influential in their own communities. Therefore, it was imperative to bring out what people wanted to talk about into the discussion without reducing their views to a generalized set of numbers to provide legitimacy to what they were saying. In the initial report for ASCI we tried to include many extracts from our interviews. But, of course, there were physical limits to this in the report. By relying on these interviews at the end, in the autumn of 2008, the research concluded that there are a number of implications of conflict processes in shaping the nature of HIV/AIDS epidemic in the country, such as changing gender hierarchy, sexual behavior and sexual violence, as well as the creation of further constraints on women's access to livelihood resources. While the research argued that there is a link between the conflict and HIV/AIDS in Burundi, the research proposed that this is not as straightforward a link as is commonly articulated within the literature on security and HIV/AIDS. The relationship is influenced by existing socio-cultural differences within a society, including race, ethnicity and religion, and determined by gender and age differences within communities. The summary of conclusions included the following:

1 There is a link between the conflict and the spread of HIV in Burundi.
2 The particular characteristics and the resolution of the conflict influence the way the HIV/AIDS epidemic is addressed in the post-conflict context.
3 Both of these processes are framed by the particular gender context in Burundi.
4 This can only be understood by looking at the gender norms and values in Burundi before the conflict, during the conflict and how they are being reconfigured in the post-conflict period.

The book

These conclusions are still relevant. However, in reconsidering the data collected in this process and reflecting on the international security discourse since the autumn of 2008 after submitting the research report to ASCI, I came to realize that these conclusions are limited within a broader framework of the research which is cast as a set of concerns on international security. The framework that was ultimately to overcome the knowledge gap in dealing with the security–HIV/AIDS link was implicitly referenced to inform international security policy. As a result, there were limits to its critical engagement. In thinking about the research material over time and in observing the way the international HIV/AIDS policy discussion has developed, it became clear that the research leading to this book provided insights for much broader questions about the way the international politics of HIV/AIDS policies are framing the discussion. Therefore, this book considers the broader question of what the research says about the international policy discussion on security. The question does not give priority to the concerns of international security discussion. It is a subject-orientated question. It considers the nature of people's everyday experiences and their relationship with HIV vulnerabilities. It then reflects on what these experiences mean for international policy thinking.

This broad question allows two analytical spaces to emerge. One is that it allows consideration of international security discussions to emerge from the overall international HIV/AIDS policy context. As I discussed in my earlier book, the initial reaction of the international policy context was to frame international HIV/AIDS as an emergency problem following existing health emergency models (2008). This was then followed by a model focusing on development processes that considered HIV/AIDS problems within international development policy frameworks. In the last decade the international security framework has become the third broad policy framework through which international HIV/AIDS policies have been articulated. While it is possible to make this analytical division between various frameworks that inform policy, in practice they interact with each other within international policy discussions. Two, the question turns the thinking about HIV/AIDS on its head, valorizing people's experiences and their perceptions about themselves and others in the context of conflict and HIV/AIDS, to think about policies that are targeting them. The approach was developed in my earlier work on knowledge claims that are based on statements of 'we know what works' (2008). The move is an epistemological shift to raise questions about the knowledge claims that are underwriting international policy discussions in relation to conflict contexts. It is also a reaction to what Didier Fassin (2007) calls 'Political anesthesia'. He describes it as the feeling we have that 'we do not feel we need to know any more than we already know' (2007: xii). In this case he is reacting to the way AIDS in South Africa is approached '[w]e have read or heard that in South Africa AIDS is a problem of sexual behaviors and peculiar beliefs' (2007: xii–xiv). The argument is about the way others become fragmentary and generic in our understanding of their problems: 'the fragmentary information we receive from an absolute elsewhere is enough for us because it confirms our sense that cultures are incommensurable and more radically social worlds are incommensurable' (2007: xiii). He is pointing out the way people lose specificity in their life contexts and become policy targets as generic groups that are in need of our help under some generic category. He adds that 'there is no inequality more disturbing than that by which we decide what is interesting and what is not, who can still interest us and who no longer does' (2007: xiii). The highlighted inequality is about how people's voices and the complexities of their lives disappear from the discussions and concerns of, in our case, policy makers and experts. People appear under a category of concern. Policy experts determine what matters in people's lives for their attention, for intervening to deal with HIV. However, when lives are categorized they are abstracted from complex lives with their particular histories, histories of engaging with disease and with each other. These are now seen through the lens of the expert who is concerned about development, security or some other issue. For my purposes this means that different people, their lives and experiences of conflict and HIV are filtered under the policy makers gaze into a limited number of security concerns. I come back to this later in the book. Here it is important to emphasize that this process not only raises questions about the ethical relationship experts and policy makers have with people and their lives, but it also points out that there are severe implications for policies that are based on partial understanding of people's lives. Experts might have divergent interests. They might only focus on those areas of people's experiences according to these interests. This situation misses the point that for people their problems are experiences that are approached in the wholeness of their lives in a particular socio-cultural and political context. Compartmentalization of these complex lives into segments based on policy interests is bound to produce significantly distorted knowledge and policies. Furthermore, this approach will undermine effective and efficacious interventions that are central to the interest of the policy makers. I agree with Fassin when he insists that 'otherness must [thus] be taken seriously. We must strive to grasp representations, practices and social facts themselves as inscribed in local history and apprehended by local actors' (2007: xiv). In order to be able to understand the intersections between conflict and HIV/AIDS the entire context needs to be understood from different positions people experience, understand and relate to these processes.

This approach then challenges the way the relationship between conflict and HIV/AIDS is framed in international security concerns. Furthermore, this move towards everyday knowledge claims has important implications for policy thinking in general. It aims to disrupt a policy process primarily determined by expert knowledge that is framing policy priorities. One way to motivate this move is to ask: What is the relevant knowledge to deal with HIV/AIDS issues in countries which are or were in conflict? Another question is: What is effective intervention? These questions shift the focus to people's experiences of HIV/AIDS in a conflict context. It also prioritizes attention to the particularities of HIV ahead of what we need to know about international security concerns.

Here I also want to highlight the position of gender in this analysis. One of the reviewers of the book proposal pointed out that my approach was finding fault with other analysts for not thinking gender important. He then suggested that I was making the opposite error: to assume the importance of gender relations before the evidence had been considered. I think this is an important issue to address. The move I mention above, towards everyday experiences and the way HIV/AIDS intersects with these everyday lives is the framing concern. The relevance of gender can be seen by considering the way the disease seems to spread. According to the Joint UN Program on HIV/AIDS (UNAIDS)'s Global Report 2010 'Slightly more than half of all people living with HIV are women and girls. In sub-Saharan Africa, more women than men are living with HIV, and young women aged 15–24 years are as much as eight times more likely than men to be HIV+' (2010: 10). The same report indicates that around 60 percent of all HIV+ people in sub-Saharan Africa are women (2010: 25). Furthermore, it points out that the majority of those newly infected with HIV in the region are infected during unprotected heterosexual intercourse (including paid sex) and onward transmission of HIV to newborns and breastfed babies (2010: 30). These considerations highlight a number of things about HIV: the primary mechanism of spread remains sexual in sub-Saharan Africa; it is generally heterosexual transmission, though same-sex transmission is also important. High levels of infected women also suggest that they are more vulnerable to the disease. This vulnerability is not only biological but related to the women's unequal power position in communities and in sexual relations (UNAIDS 2008; Campbell *et al*. 2009; Susser 2009; Gibbs 2010; Mannell 2010). Considered from this particular position, gender values and norms are a central mechanism in how the disease is spreading and impacting people's lives.

People's sexual relations are mediated according to the gender norms and values in their communities. My approach engages with the historical and sociological context of dynamic gender relations as they frame people's experiences and agency (Cockburn 1998; Puechguirbal 2010). If one wants to know what the relevant knowledge is and to produce policies that deal with HIV in people's lives, the gender context of these lives and people's attitudes are central to this knowledge to inform thinking on HIV in a given social context. The aim of the book is to think about conditions for more ethical, relevant and effective policy. Furthermore, many HIV/AIDS policy interventions are trying to initiate and influence behavior change within communities and people's lives. In people's sexual behavior, gender norms act as grounding mechanisms and set the grounds from which behavior change is a possibility. In other words, if you want individuals to change behavior you need to understand them.

In this way, gender analytical orientation is central to broader HIV/AIDS concerns. As pointed out by Lene Hansen and Louise Olsson 'to see AIDS as [a] gendered security problem implies that risks to which individual women are exposed might be situated inside an understanding of local and regional norms about sexual behavior, responsibility' (2004: 406). It provides a much broader critical analysis of the epistemological issues legitimating the top-down analysis provided in international security discussions. In other words, while the conclusions of the initial research were and are still relevant, the analysis need to go beyond the concerns of the framing question to consider the link between international security and HIV/AIDS. The gender analysis does this by locating the analysis into the socio-political context of people's lives and in explicitly questioning the relevance of the international security framework for understanding the relationship between conflict and IIIV/AIDS.

Questions on the linking of HIV/AIDS to security

The formal securitization of HIV/AIDS is a function of its inclusion in the United Nations Security Council's agenda on 10 January 2000 and the subsequent Security Council resolution related to HIV/AIDS (UN 2000). I agree with Dennis Altman (2011) that the HIV/AIDS literature developed around the questions of security presents a mature debate where a generally agreed hypothesis is developed in relation to the perceived link and this then has generated counter-arguments which have led to the reconsideration of the way HIV/AIDS has been securitized (CNN 2000; Yeager *et al.* 2000; Singer 2002; USIP 2001; Bratt 2002; Elbe 2002; Liotta 2002; Ostergard 2002; Tripodi and Patel 2002; Altman 2003; Blanchard 2003; Heymann 2003; Pistorius *et al.* 2003; UNAIDS 2003; Barnett and Prins 2005, Whiteside *et al.* 2006; Elbe 2009; McInnes and Rushton 2010). I have extensively reviewed the earlier securitization of HIV/AIDS elsewhere and will only focus on the recent discussion here (Seckinelgin *et al.* 2010).

The initial top-down securitization of HIV/AIDS is very directly questioned in an article published by Alan Whiteside, Alex De Waal and Tsadkan Gebre-Tansae in 2006. This is an important intervention as the article's title suggested the authors were revisiting some of the discussions developed in relation to HIV/AIDS and conflict. They immediately target the way assumptions were developed in this field: 'Most analyses of AIDS and national security appear to consist largely of a catalogue of reasons why the epidemic may lead to all kinds of crisis' (2006: 214). They then warn against facile causal links established in this debate on unfounded assumptions 'we can begin to dismiss some of the scenarios that have been put forward while cautioning that the epidemic's impacts on the functioning of societies are indeed its greatest security threat. Those who write on AIDS and security are advised to avoid, if at all possible, using the word 'may' or at least to note that while the epidemic may do x, it may also not do x' (2006: 215). They review foundational claims about the links between security and HIV/AIDS as mediated by conflict, soldiers, their recruitment and soldiers' field behavior. They argue that 'the oft-cited claim that soldiers have prevalence rates two to five times higher than the civilian population is unsustainable and should no longer be cited'(2006: 216). It is also argued that:

> there is remarkably little good evidence for conflict accelerating the spread of HIV/AIDS. Researchers need to disaggregate the factors in conflicts that lead on occasion to increased vulnerability to HIV and on other occasions to lesser vulnerability. Post-conflict transitions emerge as an important nexus in which vulnerability is likely to be increased.
>
> (Whiteside *et al.* 2006: 217)

This is an important statement questioning the knowledge base that led to the assumed links between security and HIV/AIDS. It is calling for evidence to establish what might be a more complicated and sociologically grounded relationship between conflict and HIV/AIDS that had not been considered so far because of the focus on military and national security. Arguably here they are implicitly critical of the debate developed up to that point within the international policy context. They point to the larger sociological context of the possible relationships in the conflict context (2006: 217). Thus they argue that the assumption which fuelled the debate from its inception and brought together many security scholars together, namely that HIV/AIDS might lead to a possible state failure, is not substantiated. Their conclusion that they 'can be sceptical about the assertion that conflict contributes to the spread of HIV and that HIV contributes to conflict' seems to suggest that they are skeptical of a particular kind of discussion that dominated the field.

Another important and searching contribution to the debate is by Stefan Elbe in his *Virus Alert* (2009). This is interesting in a number of ways as Elbe was one of the earlier scholars to participate in the development of the security–HIV/AIDS discussion with rather strong views on high infection rates and the possibilities of state failure. The book presents a different picture from his earlier arguments. In it he looks at the way HIV/AIDS was securitized and the implications this has for the disease. At this basic level the discussion is a critical review of the literature asserting a link between security and HIV/AIDS. The evidential sources of this link are questioned, and he concludes that:

> although the case in favor of considering HIV/AIDS a human security issue is robust, arguments claiming that HIV/AIDS is a national and international security threat traverse quite complex analytical terrain and are much more difficult to corroborate empirically than is usually assumed in the literature.
>
> (Elbe 2009: 55)

He then points to an important practical policy issue: 'at present there is clearly a considerable disjuncture between the weak nature of the empirical evidence base and the fervor with which policy makers are seeking to reposition HIV/AIDS as a security issue' (2009: 56). Elbe's analysis throughout the book considers a number of processes in the securitization of HIV/AIDS. For instance, he argues that this insistence within international policy-making circles is an indication of a general interest:

> those advancing the securitisation of HIV/AIDS are deliberately attempting to use the rhetorical power and connotations of security in order to increase political support and resources for international initiatives seeking to reduce the spread of HIV/AIDS among populations.
>
> (Elbe 2006: 56)

Another interesting discussion he provides is in relation to 'the transgeressive function' of sccuritization in developing countries. He argues that 'in a context where a widespread and stigmatized disease remains largely ignored by governments in the developing world, the primary concern of many working in the international politics of HIV/AIDS understandably is not a fear of excessive state mobilisation' and that:

> the language of national security—with its connotations of immediacy and urgency—is deemed to perform a useful transgressive function in terms of breaking down the wall of silence. If HIV/AIDS is a threat to national security, governments can no longer afford to ignore it.
>
> (Elbe 2009: 97)

If one puts aside the rather vague references to the developing world, the nature of stigmatization and the way governments may, or may not, be responding to HIV, there is a problem here.

This approach in Elbe's book presents a cost–benefit analysis in relation to benefit that might accrue to people in this securitization process (2009: 98–107). However, the question who decides what will be beneficial for whom given that people and the way they are experiencing the disease in the conflict context are, by and large, missing from the discussion. In the conclusion Elbe considers a number of important problems attached to the securitization of HIV/AIDS (2009: 163–70). It is argued that while it might be problematic to approach the issue with such speed without proper deliberation 'in the past normal politics has in fact meant that very little was actually done to treat people living with HIV/AIDS in the developing countries. Normal politics, in other words meant several million new infections worldwide' (2009: 164). This calculus seems to be underwriting most of the conclusion, which also argues that the securitization of HIV/AIDS creates 'an ambivalent form of social control, but it can be a useful device for resisting some of the inequalities that characterize contemporary world politics. If HIV/AIDS is a security issue, then it is possible to insist that governments do more to help people living with HIV/AIDS' (2009: 170). Again putting the rather unclear discussion of normal politics and government aside, the overall position here seems to be a politically pragmatic one. Although the thrust of the argument appears to provide an important critical lens to review the securitization debate, in terms of HIV/AIDS it appears self-referential within that particular field. There is not much on HIV/AIDS which is used to reflect on what securitization might mean for actual people rather than populations at large. Furthermore, the grounds on which securitisation takes place seem to be left out of the book. With that, the impact of such abstract knowledge claims about security and HIV is left to inform policy on practical grounds. The questions raised about the evidential base of the link are side-stepped because of the practical use of the securitization. But if there is no sufficient robust knowledge to support policies what does it mean to use securitization for practical policy purposes? What kinds of policies will this move inform? Isn't there a further danger in allowing governments to use security imperatives to engage with their populations in conflict contexts? It seems that the practical benefits of securitization are not only turning people into generic populations but they are then located in two sets of overlapping zones of exceptions to be helped (Fassin and Pandolfi 2010). *Will* we ever hear people's voices out of these zones of exceptions which focus the attention of the international policy makers? At the end this discourse seems to determine what strategies might work for people rather than what actually happen in their lives in particular contexts.

The discussion on security and HIV/AIDS is further questioned in an article by Colin McInnes and Simon Rushton in 2010. This is an important intervention as it elaborately unpacks the process leading to the UN Security Council resolution and the securitisation of HIV/AIDS. They provide an excellent analysis of the political negations behind the scenes. They argue that:

> the desire to affect policy responses was central to the securitizing move. Presenting HIV as a security issue was not simply a recognition of the dangers the epidemic posed for societies; it was also a deliberate attempt to change the way in which the disease was thought about, leading to different possibilities for action.
>
> (McInnes and Rushton 2010: 239)

Their argument supports Elbe's view that the securitization was more or less a practical political concern. However, McInnes and Rushton also disagree with Elbe that securitization has not facilitated significant new resources for HIV/AIDS in all areas. They argue that 'in the US, [then], where over the last two decades HIV/AIDS has become deeply embedded as a security issue, there is evidence of securitization having a genuine impact on policy. The key security institutions (such as the Department of Defense, the CIA and the National Intelligence Council) recognize AIDS as being within their remit, and are taking steps to address it. Yet there has been little work demonstrating a comparable impact on the policies adopted by other countries, whose security policy institutions do not appear to have seized on the issue to the same extent' (2010: 242). They have a measured view:

> we suggest that the picture emerging is not one of there being no link between HIV/AIDS and security, but rather one indicating that we require a more nuanced understanding of this link. Moreover, we argue that the initial fears expressed over the security consequences of high HIV prevalence rates were overstated and not applicable in all circumstances. Again, what is needed is a better understanding, this time of the circumstances under which HIV can impact on national security.
>
> (McInnes and Rushton 2010: 234)

While this is still somehow concerned with state security, they recognize the complexity of the experiences of the disease and the context within which those experiences take place (2010: 234).

Both Whiteside *et al.* (2006) and McInnes and Rushton (2010) provide implicit critique of the way the debate developed in the last decade out of political expedience to help people in humanitarian crisis. They are also critical of the way thinking and research were apprehended by assumptions coming from theoretical discussions on security. In their critical approach they are not arguing against understanding the relationship between conflict and HIV/AIDS. They are in fact pointing out the importance of looking at these issues from within the wider socio-political contexts in their complexity rather than reducing them to a limited number of security interests. The way security and HIV/AIDS literature has developed should not divert attention from significant implications of various conflict processes on people's lives linked with HIV/AIDS. Furthermore, in line with the orientation to take others and their complex lives seriously, analysis should pay attention to the way people perceive their conditions in conflict and think about HIV/AIDS. Conflicts and HIV/AIDS are part of larger social processes and contexts in which everyday lives are dwelled. Therefore, it is people's experiences which will determine at the end what could be said about conflicts and HIV/AIDS. It is with this view that the rest of this book is written.

Approach and structure of the book

By considering the military and armed group contexts as the most relevant for considering the risk in relation to HIV/AIDS, the security debate ignores the everyday complexities and the way they intersect with conflict processes and HIV/AIDS. Furthermore, they ignore that these intersections lead to differentiated vulnerabilities to HIV risks in a given society depending on the particulars of people's lives. This book aims to provide an alternative way of thinking about conflict and HIV/AIDS. The research material it presents provides a way of considering people's experiences, their own reflections on their well-being within the larger socio-political context of their lives. To do this I draw on the in-depth insights provided by many people in their interviews. Many of these interviews provide accounts of people's experiences during and after the conflict and reflect on their social relations and positions within that context. The material presented here is about the micro-processes grounding and facilitating people's everyday lives. In this way the interviews provide a multilayered view of nuanced social relations in which conflict processes and HIV/AIDS issues are negotiated and renegotiated. The insights they provide raise significant questions about how the international security and HIV/AIDS discussion has developed. Furthermore, they highlight problematic relationship between the analytical framing of the discussion and the policies developed to target people in the context of a particular conflict. They question the analytical content and the methodological orientation underwriting the debate.

In reporting the research I decided to use a format that allows people's voices to emerge out of the interview material. As I mentioned before, because of the nature of the questions we approached many of our interviewees with a life-history inspired approach to let them talk about their lives. This approach created rich insights about the ways people reflect and think about their experiences of conflict, HIV/AIDS and their need to be part of a larger context. They also unpack the kinds of perspectives that inform the kinds of attitudes that have developed towards HIV/AIDS in Burundi.

One could follow different strategies to report this kind of material and to develop the argument of the book. One such strategy is observed in John M. Chernoff's two-volume study of 'the true story of a young woman in West Africa' (2003: 5). In a long introduction he introduces his approach and his motivation for engaging in this study and the implications of this life story for thinking about development. After the introduction the reader is left to engage with a story of a young woman stretching over a decade in West Africa. The story is captured through recordings Chernoff conducted with her at different times in this period and in different places depending on her movements. One of his important contributions is that 'while we are thinking about their [people in this narrative] lives, they are dealing with them' (2003: 8). So while the book might appear to be a story about this young woman, she is also telling stories about *her life*. This is of course an invitation to the reader to go beyond considering the book as a report of life histories, but also to engage with and understand the way people are dealing with their own lives and issues. In other words, it is to push the reader to recognize the agency of people who are most often portrayed as disempowered.

Another possible strategy is to deploy extracts from life history interviews to illustrate and unpack questions that are important for the research field. Here the aim is to challenge the conventional view in a given field from the way interviews produce differentiated narratives. These create the analytical categories to organize the discussion, and the interview extracts provide grounding for the argument. There are important examples of this approach. The recent book by Simon Szreter and Kate Fisher (2010) looking at the experiences of sexual life in married life between 1918 and 1963, and Matt Houlbrook's (2005) book on homosexuality in London between 1918 and 1957 are good examples. In the former, Szreter and Fisher divide their book according to various concepts and issues that were challenged and unpacked through their interviews. For example, in the first section they focus on how people thought and learned about sex before and during marriage. In the chapter on facts of life they are interested in how people learned about sex and they set out the education and legal context framing the socio-cultural process in the period in which they are interested. They then rely on interview extracts. In this way, they create a conversation between existing views of that period and the ways people reflect on their experiences. In their conclusion they point out that their work suggests much more complex relationships than assumed in the literature between emerging discourses of modern sexuality and people's experiences and the way people interpreted and deployed these discourses in their lives (2010: 385–87). Houlbrook follows a similar strategy in engaging with the personal stories and the ways those stories allow the reader to observe queer lives in London between 1918 and 1957. He begins the book with Cyril's story since it highlights a set of entry points to the overall socio-political context. Houlbrook argues that 'the book maps the geography, culture and politics of queer life in London in that period' (2005: 11). This mapping provides various issues for consideration in each chapter. Depending on the issue that is addressed in the chapter, the oral history materials are employed to create a fuller picture of how the socio-legal frameworks intersected with people's lives and how they negotiated different boundaries. In each chapter a life story is used to enter the particular discussion for that chapter and other extracts are then brought to illustrate the discussion.

In both of these books, the authors acknowledge the particularities of the oral histories they report or the places they talk about, particularly in the case of Houlbrook's book on London. Szreter and Fisher clearly state that the views they present are partial and they 'recognize that the oral histories of sexual experiences within this [their] book do not provide pure or direct empirical facts about the lives, experiences and beliefs of men and women marrying' (2010: 51). However, they insist that the issue is about the way these views are unpacking experiences to reveal 'stereotypes, communal conventions, and idealizations' (2010: 11). It is these which form perceptions and inform many people's behavior as either conformity or divergence from conventions. Here, similar to Chernoff's invitation, the interest is in the way to engage with the agency of people who interpreted the conventions of their times and how they developed responses to socio-cultural, political and legal frameworks. These views provide grounded ways of thinking about the narratives, while considering the circumstances from outside. They resist becoming detached from the narratives framing people's lives and from subsuming differentiated experiences that inform social complexity in a given period within a general narrative.

In this book, I follow a combination of strategies to engage with the interview material. Most of these are linked to the life history inspired method. I could have followed a structure similar to Szreter and Fisher's work. However, I have used this style only when the interview was based more on open-ended questions and not on a life story narrative. I use large extracts from the interviews where interviewees were talking about their lives and reflecting on the way they lived in the context of the conflict. This choice is linked with a number of analytically important issues. It was clear to me that one of the reasons people wanted to talk to us and wanted to talk about their lives was because they wanted to be heard. Therefore, using the material extensively was important. Furthermore, the narratives in the chapters make it clear people's experiences were invisible outside their immediate context. In Carolyn Nordstorm's words 'the world did not see' (2009: 63). Seeing here takes on an important operational significance, because if they are not seen they disappear from the concerns expressed at local and international policy level. As a result, people's experiences remain unspoken and unheard. Yet these experiences still inform people's attitudes and behavior in interpersonal relations. The narratives also point out that 'the social world they [people] inhabit is real. While we are thinking about their lives, they are dealing with them' (Chernoff 2003: 8). Another issue here is the importance of people's everyday lives in relation to HIV/AIDS. I think longer extracts allow the reader to see the location of these issues in people's broader life contexts and the way people engage with them. People are active participants *in their own lives*, facing difficulties and opportunities; they take decisions based on their own reflections on issues that matter to them. Their reflections on HIV/AIDS and conflict are informed by their concerns about their own wellbeing. As a result, people emerge as bearers of knowledge and agency as opposed to appearing as inactive actors who are part of a larger group, who need to be helped on the basis of a few reference points that link them to the international policy concerns.

My approach also diverges from Chernoff's in some ways. I directly analyse the issues raised in a more thematic manner on conflict and HIV/AIDS. The analysis provided is a way of thinking with, and along with, people and their experiences. This process of 'thinking along' is about analysing what interviewees' reflections are saying about their interpersonal experiences and how these are unpacking their views on conflict and HIV/AIDS. This move is about changing the way we think about relevant knowledge to deal with HIV/AIDS. It moves towards considering people's everyday interpersonal experiences in a socio-historic context. This is a relevant domain of knowledge that is important for thinking about HIV/AIDS. In contrast most of the international policy discussion engages with communities and people from an HIV/AIDS-point of view. For international policy makers HIV/AIDS is the reference point through which people become intelligible. This intelligibility means that the complexity of lives is subsumed under one-dimensional representations based on HIV/AIDS models. The narratives in this book show that HIV/AIDS needs to be considered within the broader context of people's lives. Thus, the aim here is to counter HIV/AIDS-centered knowledge with a people-centered knowledge and then to think about the implications of this switch on the way an HIV/AIDS-centered approach informs international policy processes. My analysis follows what Paul Farmer (2009: 41) terms as 'writing as an outside observer'. The analysis is an engagement with people's experiences and what they reveal about international policy frames, targeting people and the way these interventions interact with their lives. The analysis is not about making expert knowledge claims on people's lives or on how they should think about themselves in the context of post-conflict socio-political relations and HIV/AIDS. It is about the way people's observations allow me and others reading them to think about the international discourse on conflict and HIV/AIDS. It is about looking at and understanding the complex intersections of conflict and HIV in everyday lives as a part of interpersonal relations. People's experiences point towards concerns that are much broader than just HIV/AIDS. They are implicitly questioning the epistemological practices of engaging with conflict from an abstract international position and the implications of such expert knowledge on international policy processes that are impacting people's lives and wellbeing.

The structure of the book is based on understanding the way conflict and gender intersect in people's lives and the way multiple intersections also influence their engagement with HIV/AIDS. Chapter 1 presents the country and conflict context in Burundi. Furthermore, it considers the way through which gender concerns emerged from the discussions with ex-combatants. Chapter 2, on the basis of the interviews, considers the gender relations in Burundi before the conflict to understand the way in which conflict processes intersected with these relations. Then Chapter 3 focuses on the way gender relations functioned during the conflict. This chapter is followed by a discussion, in Chapter 4, of how people engaged with HIV/AIDS-related issues during the conflict. Chapter 5 then considers people's experiences of post-conflict transition to highlight the impact of the intersections of conflict and gender on people's post-conflict lives. The end of this chapter provides a comprehensive view on people's gendered experiences of conflict and the implications of these experiences for HIV/AIDS concerns. Chapter 6 changes the lens through which one considers the conflict and HIV/AIDS relationship. It focuses on an influential study considering this relationship from the position of international experts. In considering this view it is possible to see the gap between the knowledge available to people as discussed in chapters up to Chapter 6 and the international expert view. Chapter 7 then reflects on the consequences of this gap and conditions under which people's experiences are ignored. Chapter 8 once again engages with people's experiences of HIV/AIDS to reflect on the way people exercise their agency even within the constraints of conflict to deal with HIV-related problems in addition to their other concerns. In the conclusion, I articulate a number of implications based on gender analysis of HIV/AIDS and people's experiences for the way international policies are framed and articulated.

1 Context, conflict, and experiences

This chapter is in two parts. The first part provides the basic background information on Burundi and the HIV/AIDS situation there. The second part presents the contours of the argument of the book as these emerge from a set of interviews at the beginning of the research. This closer look at the contours is important as the issues interviewees brought to the discussion are important markers for thinking about the intersections of conflict with HIV/AIDS. The first part of the book does not provide an in-depth analysis of the country's long-running conflict with its constantly changing dynamics and tensions over several decades. There are excellent studies looking at the multiple causes and development of violent conflicts in the post-colonial period in the Great Lakes region of Africa within the political economy of colonialism both in general and in Burundi in particular (Chrétien 2003; Daley 2008; Lemarchand 2009). These studies highlight important intra-regional and international socio-political and economic dynamics that have influenced Burundi, Rwanda, and the Democratic Republic of Congo (previously Zaire). There is no reason to repeat these discussions here. Furthermore, many of these studies provide a generalized view of the conflicts within the larger political economy of state formation or in debates related to large ethnic groups. As a result, these exhibit a particular homogeneous view on the causes and implications of these conflicts. Sometimes the homogeneity is at the level of the country, the region, or ethnic groups. This is where this book provides an important contribution. Peter Uvin's (2009) book *Life After Violence: A People's Story of Burundi* provides similarly important insights and discussions to this debate. While there are differences between his study and the study reported here in terms of their focus and methods, Uvin's book provides significant parallel's with the present work. In contrast to the generalized outlook of the studies above, the discussion here looks at individuals and the stories of the way they have experienced the conflict and HIV/AIDS. Here, similar to Uvin's work, the way Burundi is considered is based on the people's conflict as they experienced it, rather than using comparative narratives about the region that were constructed from international security perspectives. In order to locate these experiences within the social and political context of the country, I first provide a brief overview of the conflict in Burundi.

Burundi

Burundi is 27,834 km² in area; this includes 2,000 km² of Lake Tanganyika. This country is similar in size to Belgium (30,000 km²), the Netherlands (33,700 km²), Lesotho (30,000 km²), Switzerland (41,000 km²), Albania (28,000 km²), Haiti (27,840 km²), and Rwanda (26,338 km²). Burundi is situated approximately 2,100 km from the Atlantic Ocean, and 1,100 km from the Indian Ocean. Burundi's population is approximately 8.6 million, which consists of 14 percent Tutsi, 85 percent Hutu, and 1 percent Twa.

After establishing a monarchy in the sixteenth century, Burundi became a part of German East Africa in 1899. During World War I Burundi came under Belgian rule before gaining independence in 1962. An attempted coup in 1965 led the king to flee Burundi, never to return, while refusing to abdicate. The king's son eventually took power, although it was short lived; in November 1966, Captain Michel Micombero gained power through a military coup. He abolished the monarchy and declared Burundi a republic while the king was away on an official visit.

In 1972, a Hutu rebellion killed large numbers of Tutsi. According to Chrétien (2002), 150,000 people were massacred and a larger number of people fled the country. In November 1976, Colonel Jean Baptiste Bagaza gained control through a military coup and exiled his predecessor. In September 1987, Major Pierre Buyoya of the Union for National Progress (*Union pour le Progrès national* (UPRONA)) took power for the first time, also through a military coup. Burundi faced a considerable Hutu rebellion in 1988. Here the role of the Party for the Liberation of the Hutu People (*Parti pour la libération du peuple hutu* (PALIHUTU)) was important in pushing people to violence against the Tutsi. All three of the military coups were carried out successively by high-ranking military officers originating from the Tutsi ethnic group, and from the same commune in the southern province of Bururi. In 1991 the Charter of Unity was adopted by referendum. It condemned all discrimination and exclusion and it was followed by a new constitution in 1992. Under this charter and constitution, no ethnically based political party or organization was to be registered in the country. This was significant later, for instance, for the cease fire discussions with the PALIPEHUTU FNL (National Forces of Liberation (*Forces nationales de libération*)) from 2007 onwards. They were granted provisional immunity as a signatory to the cease-fire accord with the Government on September 7 2006. As they prepared to come to Bujumbura to implement the accord, their leaders were demanding to be clearly named in the law as PALIPEHUTU FNL. And the government argued that this was against the constitution to do so.

Before 1992, nearly all ministers, civil servants, and military personnel were from the Tutsi ethnic group; people from the Hutu ethnic communities were widely excluded. All of the military coups until 1993 were perceived as strategies needed by the Tutsi to hold on to power. This created a view that the Tutsis were allied to people in the government. Moreover, Tutsi power was seen as part of the military and regionally based, since three consecutive presidents were Tutsi and came from Bururi province in the south of the country. Under these presidencies large numbers of soldiers were recruited from the Tutsi ethnic group, especially from provinces such as Bururi and Muramvya. Major Buyoya lost the presidency when Burundi held its first democratic presidential elections in 1993, as the Front for Democracy in Burundi (*Front pour la Démocratie au Burundi* (FRODEBU)) candidate Melchior Ndadaye became the first civilian and Hutu president of the country. Ndadaye was assassinated after only three months in office, which sparked the start of a civil conflict which lasted almost 13 years. His successor's time in office was also short-lived, since after only two months in the post Cyprien Ntaryamira together with the president of Rwanda died when the plane they were traveling in was shot down over Kigali, Rwanda, in April 1994. He was replaced by the speaker of the National Assembly, Sylvestre Ntibantunganya. Ntibantunganya's government established power sharing between FRODEBU and UPRONA. In June 1994 a faction in FRODEBU splintered and established the National Council for the Defense of Democracy (*Conseil National Pour la Défense de la Démocratie*)—with Forces of the Defense of Democracy (*Forces pour la Défense de la Démocratie*—(CNDD-FDD-NCDD-FDD)) as its armed wing. It was led by Leonard Nyangoma, a prominent political figure since Ndadaye's time in government. The CNDD-FDD split in 2001 and Pierre Nkurunziza became leader of the newly established faction. It established alliances with other rebel groups, PALIPEHUTU and the National Liberation Front—*Front pour la liberation nationale* (FROLINA). By March 1995, ethnic division and fighting was rife, particularly in Bujumbura. These political changes and alliances uprooted the Tutsi and reintroduced Hutus coming from neighboring countries in which they had been exiled since 1972. After the July 1996 massacre of displaced people in the rural province of Gitega, former president Buyoya retook power with the help of the military, which remained predominantly Tutsi. As a result, international actors put an embargo on the country until 1999. In the process, Buyoya managed to establish links with FRODEBU through a "convened government," allowing a certain number of Hutus to be in his cabinet.

The Arusha Peace and Reconciliation Accords for Burundi was signed in August 2000; this was a very important step in the peace process. It was agreed that there would be a 36-month transition period. This period would be divided into two halves. In October 2001, a transitional constitution was written that made this provision law: an arrangement between the G7 and the G10. During the first transition period, the country would be led by an individual from the group of 10 Tutsi political parties (G10). During the peace talks, PALIPEHUTU split into two factions, each of them claiming to be the real PALIPEHUTU. The FNL also was divided into two FNL factions. One of them (led by Dr. Karatasi) signed the Arusha accords, while the faction led by Agathon Rwasa was still fighting. FRODEBU is a mainly Hutu-based party. Sylvestre Ntibantunganya, former president of the republic, is a prominent member of this party. UPRONA is predominantly a Tutsi-based party, of which Pierre Buyoya, former president of the republic, is an influential member. Buyoya was chosen for this reason. The second period would be led by one from the group of seven Hutu political parties (G7), and Domitien Ndayizeye was chosen by the Hutu parties. Some of the small Tutsi political parties did not sign the accord immediately in Arusha. They argued that they had reservations on many issues. However, they later joined and signed the accord. However, after the accord was signed, the parties continued in discussions while war continued on the ground. It was not until late 2003 that fighting in the CNDD and FDD strongholds subsided. A power-sharing deal was negotiated and a new government was formed in December 2003 that included Pierre Nkurunziza. The FNL remained outside the ceasefire agreement and although an initial agreement was eventually signed in May 2005 it was not upheld. Thus, fighting continued and a second ceasefire agreement was eventually signed in September 2006. Fighting remained periodic until late 2008. A new constitution was passed early in 2005 and the second democratic presidential elections took place in August of the same year, with the CNDD-FDD winning overwhelmingly. Pierre Nkurunziza was sworn in as the president of the republic and the new government was installed in September 2005. The president was elected by the parliament on that occasion. The first direct elections for the presidency took place on June 28 2010, when President Nkurunziza was re-elected (HRW 2010; WFN 2010).

The Burundian administrative structure after the 2005 election

Burundi is divided into 18 provinces (including the capital Bujumbura, *Bujumbura Marie* with its 13 urban communes) each headed by a Governor nominated by the President of the Republic. The constitution of 2005 stipulated a 30 percent female quota to represent women at all levels of government. At the time of the research, four of the 18 provincial Governors were women. Provinces are divided into communes. There are 129 communes, which are governed by a communal counsel consisting of 25 people, headed by a Communal Administrator and elected directly by the inhabitants in 2005. In many communes, the CNDD-FDD party has the majority of seats in the Communal Councils. Before 2005 Communal Administrators were appointed by the President, after consultation with the Governor, and no positions were occupied by women. Now, 30 percent of the Administrators are women, whereas during the war most of the communal administrators were soldiers.

Each commune is subdivided in two to four zones. The Chief of Zone is appointed by the Governor of the Province, after consultation with the Communal Administrator. Each zone contains two or three sectors. The chief of sector is appointed by the Governor of the Province after consultation with the Communal Administrator. Each zone is divided into hillsides (*collines*). A hillside is the smallest administrative area in Burundi. There is an elected

Hillside Council which consists of up to five people: the one who receives the most votes automatically becomes the Chief of the Hillside. The country contains approximately 2,650 hillsides. Previously, below the hillside unit there were sub-hillsides and Head of 10 houses subdivisions (*Myumbakumi*). Both of the divisions were abolished under the 2005 communal law.

Here it is also important to highlight the traditional institution of the *bashingantahe*, which traces its background to the pre-colonial period. Here, I rely on Uvin's (2009: 61–66) excellent definition and description of this institution. The institution consisted of men giving judgment and advice in local conflicts. These men were elected in a community according to their standing. Importantly the institution was non-ethical and both Hutu and Tutsi could become members. However, in time, with the colonial administrations and also at present, the members were appointed from outside the community by political authority. As Uvin points out the tradition of the community nominating parts of the institution still survives as "*bashingantahe investi*" (2009: 62). While their authority is still to a degree recognized and they were mentioned by many during the interviews, the way their authority sits with the more non-traditional political administrative authority is complex. In particular, the way government's political authority interferes with the appointment process seems to have created discomfort within communities. Many people we talked to said that they were unsure whose interests the advice they would get from *bashingantahe* would serve. Uvin points out that the traditional beer drinking after the decision is transformed, and now "*bashingantahe* ask for beer before agreeing to get involved, and will make decisions in favor of the one who managed to pay them in beer" (Uvin 2009: 63). We were also told about this situation by many people, particularly women. In one of the interviews, we were told that she wanted to discuss her marriage arrangements and demand resources from her husband but she could not go to *bashingantahe* as they wanted a case of beer and she did not have money to pay for this. This suggests that the top-down appointment process arguably may have gradually changed the accountability mechanisms which linked members of *bashingantahe* more directly with their community. According to Uvin, this complication might very well be a control mechanism by the current government which:

> is wary of a corps of people with major public roles who are entirely uncontrolled ... one way to reduce the power of the bashingantahe has been the creation of deliberate confusion: the newly elected members of the "*conseil de colline*" [hillside], the lowest level of public administration are now given the title of "*elected bashingantahe*" with presumably the prerogatives as the "invested" ones.
>
> (Uvin 2009: 63–64)

It is also important to point out that, as Ndeye Sow (2006) argues, women were broadly excluded from the formal peace negotiations in the Arusha

Peace process and in the subsequent ceasefire talks between the Burundian Government and the FNL. There was a broad reluctance to recognize women's right to participate in these processes. However, with the help of international non-governmental organizations and international organizations funding the Arusha Peace process "seven women were given observer status during the negotiations" (Falch 2010: 10) and women were able to lobby for "the inclusion of 30 provisions for women in the agreement" (Sow 2006: 10). These influenced the formal participation of women in the political process in the drafting of the Accord. In the 2005 Constitutional Referendum marking the symbolic end of the conflict, the document stipulated 30 percent representation of women in Parliament. In the subsequent period, women accounted for 34 percent of the Senate and 31 percent of the National Assembly, and a woman was appointed as the Speaker of Parliament. Here the actual election process produced fewer than expected women so additional representatives were co-opted into the Senate and the Assembly (Falch 2010: 12). The outcome of these processes in terms of the ability of women politicians to influence gendered policy outcomes remains unclear.

AIDS in Burundi

According to the World Health Organization (WHO) (2005), AIDS was first diagnosed in Burundi in 1983. The organization reported a rapidly growing epidemic after that period. It estimated that at the end of 2003 "250,000 adults and children were living with HIV/AIDS and an estimated 25000 people died from AIDS during 2003" (WHO 2005). The Burundian trajectory is one of a generalized epidemic. The WHO refers to a national survey from 2002 showing HIV in the general population was 5.4 percent and that prevalence rates in urban, semiurban, and rural areas were 9.4 percent, 10.5 percent, and 2.5 percent, respectively. In 1989, the prevalence rate in urban areas was close to 11 percent, whereas the prevalence rate in rural areas was 0.7 percent. The 2002 national survey also indicated that women in urban areas were more likely to be infected than men, whereas the same proportion of men and women were infected in rural areas. The HIV seroprevalence among women attending antenatal clinics in Bujumbura (the capital) was 16 percent in 2001 (WHO 2005). According to UNAIDS estimates in 2009, in Burundi around 180,000 people are living with HIV, the adult prevalence rate is 3.3 percent, around 90,000 women are considered to be living with HIV, and there were 200,000 orphans due to AIDS (UNAIDS 2009).

Burundi followed a structured administrative path to policy delivery in relation to HIV/AIDS. The structure was underpinned, initially, by a separate Ministry responsible for HIV/AIDS which was situated directly within the office of the President of the Republic to show the political commitment of the state. In 2002 the government created the National AIDS Council (*Conseil National de Lutte contre le SIDA* (CNLS)) in line with international guidelines. From 2002 onwards the CNLS has been at the forefront of the

Burundian strategy. The Burundian strategic approach worked on the basis of a decentralization in which responsibilities were given to provinces and communes. The CNLS structure is decentralized at the level of provinces into the *Comité Provincial de Lutte contre le SIDA* (CPLS). Then this is decentralized at the level of the smaller administrative unit of communes to *Comité Communal de Lutte contre le SIDA* (COCOLS). In some cases the decentralization can also be observed at the school level, where many have Stop Sida clubs to sensitize students using a peer-education model.

The country also received international funding from the World Bank, the Global Fund, and from bilateral donors. Between 2003 and 2006 the fund provided aid through the first round under the *Renforcement de l'Initiative Burundaise dans le domaine de la Prévention et la prise en charge des PVVIH* (RIBUP) project. Then, during the fifth round it provided funding of US$32 million for 2006–11 under *Appui au Programme d'Intensification et de la Décentralisation de la lutte contre le VIH/SIDA au Burundi* (APRODIS) project. The projects were focusing on risk reduction, sensitization of people, and other prevention-related activities as well as the provision of ant-retroviral therapy (ART) for those in need. In addition to various international non-governmental organizations working in Burundi on HIV/AIDS, there are two important national organizations: the Burundi Network of People Living with HIV and AIDS (*le Réseau Burundais des Personnes vivant avec le VIH* (RBP+)) and the National Association for the Support of Seropositive and people affected by AIDS (*l'Association Nationale de soutien aux Seropositifs et Malades du Sida* (ANSS)). Both of these organizations are working on advocacy for people infected and affected by HIV/AIDS and to deliver services to people ranging from care to treatment. They also receive funding through CNLS from international donors. The main international funders for HIV/AIDS are international donors, and both multilateral and bilateral aid play a significant role for Burundi. The multilateral actors include the World Bank and The Global Fund to Fight AIDS, Tuberculosis and Malaria.

However, relations between donors and the government of Burundi are not always very straightforward. For instance, in December 2007 in Burundi a statement by the president on international AIDS day caught many people's attention. On that occasion he was very severe and direct in his speech. President Pierre Nkurunziza stated that:

> Donors' failure to help Burundi fight against HIV/AIDS and bring support to patients is a simple genocide they will be held responsible for. We cannot accept that people keep dying for lack of medicines, while in other countries they are getting assistance.

This was a response to a policy decision taken by the Global Fund in November 2007. At the time, a spokeswoman for the Global Fund announced that:

Burundi's proposal in Round 7 had been unsuccessful and the Fund's technical review panel had informed the country coordinating mechanism of their decision. Burundi submitted a proposal requesting more than US $95 million over a five-year period for HIV/AIDS and TB, but the technical review panel found that the application had not adequately addressed the feasibility of implementing the grant.

(IRIN 2007)

This was frustrating for many people living with the disease and those who were trying to implement interventions to deal with the disease in the country. As reported by health officials in Bujumbura at the time: "nearly 6,000 people will be short of life-prolonging antiretroviral (ARV) drugs in 2008. An estimated 10,000 people were accessing ARVs in December 2007, out of an estimated 50,000 who need the drugs" (IRIN 2007). Dr. Jean Rirangira, technical director of CNLS, identified a shortfall "of US$11 million of the total of $28 million required to fight the pandemic" in 2008 (IRIN 2007). The net impact of this shortfall led the government to reconsider its plans, "as voluntary counseling and testing centers could not be scaled up as planned, and funding for income-generating activities for people affected by AIDS would have to be curtailed" (IRIN 2007). Burundi, similar to many low-income countries, relies heavily on international aid to deal with HIV/AIDS. Any change in international policy frameworks informing aid relations creates complex challenges both for people living with the disease and for those who are trying to deliver resources to them in the country. The following reflections highlight this problem.

Responding to a question about the announcement of no funding by the Global Fund in November 2007, a senior health specialist stated that "it will be a catastrophe! There will be need for buying lots of coffins. There are 9000 people under ARV treatment" (IRIN 2007). One year later in October 2008, nearly a year after the decision, Dr. Jean Rirangira, who was now the interim executive secretary of CNLS, said that "it has been very hard; we have tried to use our internal resources and prioritise interventions to make sure that we cover the most important activities." She added:

we have continued to buy ARVs and train a few doctors, but our prevention efforts and attempts to help orphans and vulnerable children have suffered. We had plans to expand services for prevention of mother-to-child transmission [PMTCT] of HIV, but we have had to postpone them till we get more funding.

(IRIN 2008)

The situation was described by the ANSS, which had benefited from the Global Fund and had a large ART delivery program, as:

access to ARVs is now limited to people whom we were already supplying, and their families. In addition to drugs, if we wanted to maintain the quality of service that we provide, we would need to train and hire more doctors. Right now, our four doctors see 20 patients each per day and we don't want to overload them, so we cannot expand.

(IRIN 2008)

In October 2008 it was announced that the Global Fund's Technical Review Panel decided to recommend that Burundi's application for funds from the eighth round of grants, amounting to US$150 million over five years, be accepted. In 2010 treatment issues have also become complicated as "the National AIDS Control Council (CNLS) finalized its agreement with RBP+ facilitating the delivery of free medical care which reached an estimated 22,000 members of the RBP+. Under the system, members are issued with cards entitling them to free treatment, which is then billed to RBP+" (AC 2010). According to Déo Kameya, the head of the RBP+ branch in the eastern province of Rutana, "out of 500 registered HIV-positive people in the area, about 350 now had to provide for their own medical care." He added that "If a person living with HIV goes to the hospital for medical care and receives a prescription, if he can afford the price of medicines it is ok, if not, he simply dies." He also said. "At present we have nowhere to [go] to get support for them" (IRIN 2010). Rose Nyandwi, health coordinator in the northern province of Ngozi, said people in her province could not afford the tests required to determine eligibility for ARVs: "We direct them to do tests but sometimes we wait for them to bring back results in vain. With such low CD4 counts [a measure of immunity] as 50 or 100 … they stay home and die" (IRIN 2010). The tensions evident in these views frame the kind of environment that frames people's post-conflict experiences with the disease.

Contours of people's conflict

Our research began with a long discussion among the researchers about the difficulties of asking questions about the conflict and the similar difficulties of asking questions about HIV/AIDS in Burundi. This was a major constraint since the questions used to lead the interviews and the discussion had to be constantly reconsidered. The main concern was not to retraumatize participants by engaging with them in an inappropriate manner (Uvin 2009). However, some of these carefully designed questions were thrown out at the first meeting in a discussion with three ex-combatants. Their responses to the questions were very open and direct.

In this section I focus on this discussion, as it highlights major tensions about HIV/AIDS both in the conflict and in the post-conflict contexts. The lines of analysis that emerge from this discussion are important since they underline the main pathways for understanding the relationship between conflict and HIV/AIDS as it matters to people living in that context.

The three interviewees were all ex-combatants. They were of different ages and represented different aspects of the rebellion. One was from the regular

Burundian Army during the conflict (FAB) and he had also been a communal administrator during the same period (A). He was 50 and married at the time of the interview. The other two participants were from one of the main rebel groups which had been in the government since the end of the conflict CNDD-FDD. B was 40 and married at the time of the interview. The last participant was around 13 when he joined the rebellion and thus was a child soldier during the conflict (C). At the time of the interview he was 18, an orphan, without land and looking after his older sister who was ill. At the end of the conflict and through the disarmament process he was still under-age. He had refused to demobilize under the child-soldier program. All three interviewees were representing a group of ex-combatants in their own areas. They were acting as local points of contact for various administrative authorities within the reintegration and reinsertion process.

The interview aimed to understand the views on the way conflict and HIV had interacted and also how gender positions were instrumental in these relations. We began the discussion by considering whether they knew much about HIV/AIDS during the conflict.

c: FAB and rebels were affected. I saw and was part of regular rebel sexual abuses, and heard many military rapes. I believe women have no voice. We had no radio to hear news about it [HIV] and now we [excombatants] have no groups helping us.

a: HIV is not visible both now and during the conflict due to three reasons: There were no testing opportunities; lack of training in dealing with HIV or information on HIV and today we are not invited to seminars on HIV; people are also afraid to be tested—are afraid of being laughed at or humiliated. I believe training would help and tests allow people to organize their lives.

c: I was in the bush for 6 years (18 at the time of the interview), I am afraid of HIV testing and have not yet tested. I need to discuss with people who are knowledgeable–maybe then ... I saw many difficult things. I kidnapped girls, raped them (what happened to those girls?) they became soldiers. Some could became your girlfriend ... some were kidnapped from their villages and subsequently trained and remained in the rebellion, some wanted to join. ... I see lots of sex in Kamenge [section of suburban Bujumbura] now.

b: I saw bad things. We were given orders to rape women. We called these women "akarago" [mats for beds]. I saw that I have been part of it. I did this 4 or 5 times I did not use condoms. Combatants did so (these acts) because they were energized. I think many excombatants are infected ... Both men and women were combatants ... some were "married," both fought, they may or may not be demobilized together ... Many would like more sensitization, information of protection and how to stop the spread. Excombatant behavior has not changed.

a: Young people from rural areas come to urban areas to use sex-workers. They [young and excombatants] are not invited to meetings [sensitization sessions] on HIV. It is because government decides the participants; the communal administrator finalizes the list and decides not to include excombatants.

All three agreed that there was no HIV information in the forces or in the bush where the rebels were. Most of the information was about ethnicity and not about HIV. They also thought that the demobilization program in the demobilization camps were too short; they felt that it needed to be repeated many times to be internalized, especially since they were in such a state of shock and preparing to be reintegrated into their communities.

INTERVIEWER: Could you speak openly about HIV during this period or after the camps?

B: We now could but we need more information and it needs to be repeated.

C: The battalion ordered rapes, kidnapping—girls especially for officers. Officers used to order their troops to kidnap young women for them.

A: In IDP camps where the military was ordered to protect its inhabitants, the soldiers often assaulted women, especially widows, many widows. They knew that the women had no mechanism to complain so they could get away with it. I saw HIV spread in these camps.

C: Many women would be kidnapped and raped, they lived with armed groups as "wives," we just "took women," especially when drunk, we did not know them, there was lots of sex.

B: After demobilization, people avoided excombatants and it was hard to get married (especially in the first year) we were seen as animals.

INTERVIEWER: What was it like to come back/returning home?

A: It was a question of trust—women[wives] were obliged to trust the men. They knew that men had sex while away but the women just had to trust them [it is not the women's choice to defy their husband even under these circumstances], both men and women had sex when their partners were absent.

C: I have a friend (rebel) with children, during the conflict he never saw them (1998–2000) but now live together.

B: Some wives [whose husbands were in the rebellion] went to IDP camps or cities, the fighters tried to visit as often as they could but often the elapsed time was enormous, officers had other relations outside the marriage.

INTERVIEWER: Were wives given the responsibility for the house when the men were away?

C: Officers in the FAB were given opportunities to go home to visit families. This allowed for joint organization, decision in the house. In the rural areas, the women were forced to be responsible for all household duties. Fighters never saw their families and this is why they had sexual relations in the bush. They could have sex with different women on many different occasions.

INTERVIEWER: Are soldiers better informed about HIV now?

C: No, not really.

B: Depends on the government: Now the FDN seems to be better equipped and is fighting HIV. In schools there is information, but with excombatants, no. ...

A: In 1984–93 there were sessions on HIV (in the military) but from 1993 until the end of the crisis they ceased. People in the bush received no training, had widespread unprotected sex. Now it is better.

C: Not yet tested for HIV, I am still fearful but have had conversations about it. Conversation like this (the interview) really helps.

B: Many Burundians are fearful, they fear to be tested; they need open forums to discuss, not just to test ... many feel that if their children remain healthy over the years, then both the children and themselves are free from HIV—this is their "HIV testing mechanism."

A: Testing is a good idea, discussions say two times per month would be good to help convince people to be tested.

INTERVIEWER: Do you think condom use is important?

A: In Burundi, and in other places, people are ashamed to use condoms, ashamed to buy them in public, soldiers have them in dispensers but are cautious that people will see them take condoms. They know that sex workers have them.

B: Some people had condoms but they were kept in pockets or wallets and the bad storage made them unusable. Many men looked at women and judged their health by their appearance; if they looked healthy; they were deemed to be healthy and could have sexual relations with them easily.

A: Women cannot ask for condoms, and rural women absolutely Not. Alcohol played a huge part in sex, if drunk, men, did not think to use condoms, rural women would be ashamed, no freedom to ask for condoms and negotiate sex.

B: [Women] only used [condoms] if men insisted, men are afraid of female condoms, easier for a woman to have choices if she was educated, rural women did not have the notion of condoms in their minds, rural women never asked to use condoms.

C: If women had education they were more likely to speak out.

INTERVIEWER: How was the reintegration?

C: Relations were good, no conflict.

A: That is a hard question—in the Burundian custom, wife must obey and respect husband, therefore, she must welcome him without any issues, that was tradition-women had no decision making ability.

B: I saw problems, especially if the man was away for prolonged periods of time, 5 years, it is difficult for a woman. It was hard especially if they had a child with someone-this cause separation and divorce. Sometimes the man had children as well and brought them home, causing tension, there is an issue of mistreatment of these children by the wife.

A: In the population they (rebels and FAB soldiers) were welcomed differently because the population were told that FAB was there to "protect" them whereas rebels were their enemy. There was different language used for the different groups of fighters. Therefore, it was hard for average people to treat excombatants—the population was unwelcoming. There were no resources, jobs and people were afraid that relations would not be peaceful.

C: There were different treatment and perceptions amongst FAB and rebel forces—it was the first time they were not fighting each other, that there was peace amongst them. When they entered FDN relations were not great, no sharing of food at the beginning, but after, it was better.

At the end of the interview there was a period where the discussion carried on more informally. For instance, C talked about how at the end of the day he thought it was better to be part of a group rather than be in the middle of fighting and pushed around by different groups. According to him, independent of his very bad experience, he was still safer among the rebel group. This was also confirmed by others who agreed with him. C also talked about his cross-country travels how he initially was sent to the eastern Congo (Democratic Republic of Congo (DRC)) where he was trained and then joined his group back in Burundi. Both B and C talked about their movements between Burundi and neighboring countries such as Tanzania and the DRC. An interesting aspect of this discussion was the ease with which A, who was from the FAB, participated and discussed these movements with them. The interview process produced two important issues. It was clear that independent of their differences and fighting history ex-combatants shared common ground. This is linked to the way they become "ex" through the demobilization and reinsertion processes. While it was clear that they did not have time to think too much about the other side while fighting in the conflict, the demobilization process brought the different groups together. Furthermore, the challenges of demobilization and reinsertion also represented a problem about how men in arms relate to civilian life. In the present case this was severe yet also nuanced. While many of the rebels lived in the bush for long periods of time, considering the nature and the duration of the conflict they were not always separated from civilians; in fact they were in a constant relationship with the civilian population. As the interviewees made clear, it was the nature of this relationship that made reinsertion much harder. The shared experience which could be observed in the discussion is also about forging new relations and becoming a part of their communities.

This interview process also demonstrated that the assumption about people's reticence to discuss the conflict or HIV/AIDS was not accurate. All three were very open about their experiences and their thinking around these issues. They discussed rather violent episodes from their experiences and reflected on the reasons why they found themselves in those situations, and this was difficult for us to listen to. It was not clear what was the correct reaction when sexual violence from the past was mentioned. These revelations were unexpected and were not solicited with direct questions on sexual violence. The immediate reaction one felt was not limited to the fact that these were potentially criminal cases. One also felt confused in terms of how to engage with them: should I stop the interview and give them a short but sharp dressing down or should I just ignore what is being said and come to terms with it after the interview? While thinking about these it was impossible to ignore the tone in which the discussion was taking shape. Both B and C were clearly unhappy about their past. They presented themselves as victims of higher ranks and the circumstances. This was, however, not a way of absolving themselves from responsibility. It was clear that they felt responsible for their actions. More importantly, they were trying to come to terms with how these events from their past had important implications for their present. C was physically uncomfortable with his own words but wanted to discuss it further. He was reflecting on the fact that such sexual violence now haunts him in his everyday life. He said that "I have a girlfriend and we want to marry but how could I? I am not even sure I am HIV or not? I must have it." It is also clear from in B's remark above when he described being considered as animals after the conflict while they were trying to reintegrate. This was a self-reflection as he thought their own behavior was unacceptable and was most of the time forced. He said that they were asked to engage in these violent acts to show their strength as men and as a member of a particular group. In other words, sexual violence was used as a demonstration of loyalty and belonging. Given the reasons why C joined the rebellion and his age at the time not joining in would have created a dangerous situation for him. His actions, therefore, were not entirely irrational though he stated that most of the time they were also drunk. The violent interaction seems to, in this case, indicate a self-preservation instinct. This particular point about taking a difficult decision to survive is made later in the research in other places in Burundi too.

While at the time it was hard to assess how common these experiences were, it was clear that they were relating to unhappy and traumatizing experiences for them. Of course, in the post-conflict context they are now living ordinary lives, but they were also very sensitive to the conditions of women, and it was this sensitivity which was channeling their reflections on the women they had met in the past. C was reflecting on his girlfriend while B was talking about his wife. Their comments reported above in relation to women also show this sensitivity, which is the result of trying to come to terms with what happened during the conflict and how they were personally involved in these violent episodes. When they are talking about women's voicelessness, it is clear that this is based on their experience of engaging with women where they did not actually care how women were reacting to the violence. It is also interesting that they seemed to think that the disempowerment of women was linked to lack of education. However, A responded with disbelief when asked whether women could decide the number of children they wanted and whether they wanted to use condoms. His response was a categorical *no*, independent of the education women might have. The common feeling within the discussion was that they needed more space to discuss and think about their experiences. When asked whether they had been given any such space to share these reflections since the end of the conflict, the response was *no*, they didn't have space to discuss these issues. Furthermore, they also mentioned that now after the conflict *no one wanted to know what happened during to conflict*. They were never asked about their experiences once they came out of the conflict; now they were expected to reintegrate and get on with their lives. Here in these reflections they were resentful of the system as they thought the experiences that they had shared with us had important implications for their lives, but that they were unable to engage with these.

These discussions taken in their entirety still require one to think how to engage with the interviewees. What is the role of the researcher when unexpected information emerges from the research process? There is no easy answer to this question. Their reflections on their conditions and their very open approach to their own past in terms of their present condition were educational. It was also clear that they took the interview as an opportunity to engage with each other and with themselves and use it to come to terms, in the case of C, for instance, with possible HIV status. The openness of these interviewees was unexpected, and informed how we had to approach others in the overall research. The first interview session meant that we had to reconsider our interview style and introduce an approach that was more inspired by the oral history method. This was to let people speak and reflect on their experiences. It was clear from this experience that people had not been given space to talk about their experiences. Therefore, it was important to use the space provided by interviews for a more engaging exercise. The research was interested in people's experiences and their reflections; if they wanted to use this space and the questions themselves to reflect on the past that was fine. This approach provided a pragmatic solution in terms of the research and how one would approach the information we were hearing. The approach allowed us to consider the unexpected to be located in the context of one's life experience over a period of time and also allowed us to think about the interviewee's own reflections in relation to these issues.

Thinking about these discussions has been a long-term engagement since the end of the research. It has required going back to the interview material and reflecting both on what is being said and on the process as a part of the information that it has generated. What did it mean to talk about these issues for the people participating in this process? Why did they share this information? What is the role of such reflections on thinking about this information? No doubt people's own reasons to engage in the research and to discuss their experiences need to be part of the way one thinks about the information. Their intention to use the interview as an occasion to reflect on their experiences demonstrates a process of internal questioning. It is possible to consider that individuals are stuck between their experiences and the perspective of many communities, which in the words of B, consider them to be animals.

They are not given any space to talk about their experiences and to reflect on their implications. Even if they think about these experiences internally, as could be ascertained from the above interview material, it is difficult to come to terms with these experiences discursively. According to the discussion this then leads to silences and difficulty in changing behavior. Here the individual voices challenge the categorical approach to perpetrators of sexual violence and rape during conflicts. However, the challenge is not about ambivalence towards such acts, they are unacceptable. There is no doubt these acts are criminal offenses against humanity. The challenge is about the perpetrators: how to think about perpetrators of such acts as human beings. Furthermore, it is about how the perpetrators need to be addressed in post-conflict contexts. Should they be prosecuted or persecuted? Do they have a right to be rehabilitated? This question is, of course, linked with a broader question of how far they are considered to be part of the community and thus a part of the future of that society. Furthermore, is there a need to have a balance between punishment and rehabilitation in societies which have already been destabilized by longer term conflict? Scott Atran in his work looking at terrorist groups and their violent extremism argues that "understanding small-group dynamics can trump individual personality" (2010: 223). I think there is an analogy here, at least in so far as the group dynamics are concerned, in influencing individuals to commit sexual violence. However, it is also important to consider how the cognitive world of groups is related with the individual's actions to produce such results. It is imperative to consider structures and processes that influence ordinary people to commit these kinds of acts which would be impossible for them under normal circumstances. In the conflict context attitudes that instrumentalize women's (and in some contexts men's) bodies need to be part of the thinking on the mechanism behind these behaviors. The argument here also points out that by dealing with individuals and punishing those individuals for atrocities, justice is seen to be done. Individuals could be prosecuted and punished for their actions. However, it is not always clear whether this justice then leads to behavioral and structural changes that influence people's actions and that led to the sexual violence and rape.

Why do these interviews matter?

On reflection, the first set of interviews reported above came to provide direction for the issues that inform this book and its analysis. The main interest of the research was to understand, as I stated in the introduction, how HIV/AIDS interacted with the conflict and how these interactions were addressed in post-conflict Burundi. This research aimed to contribute to the larger debate on the relationship between security and HIV/AIDS. Here security is cast broadly as an international concern often related to some form of trouble with a state which will have ramifications for regional or international peace. So what does the above reported discussion have to say about this issue? Admittedly, from this perspective it does not say much. It reports a discussion among three ex-combatants in a long conflict. It is hard to deduce any strong analytical contributions these might make to the international security debate. However, they do say something more remarkable. They change the perspective on the discussion about HIV and conflict.

The discussion above highlights a set of risks and risky behavior in relation to the ex-combatants and the way their lives were structured during the conflict. To look at them, without getting involved with a deep discussion at this stage, suggests that some of these risks are linked with the differentiated nature of the armed groups. These were also linked to the different position's individuals had within the armed groups, in addition to reflecting on how armed groups were linked and engaged with different communities. I am intentionally not using the language of civilians as being a civilian and being a part of the rebellion were interchangeable attributes at different times. Insecurity in relation to HIV was a function of one's social context that is defined according to different markers in the conflict. On the whole, however, the risks were generated by sexual activity. And the nature of sexual relations was clearly influenced by the nature of the conflict. This includes its duration, and its patterns of dislocation.

While these insecurities are highlighted, the discussion also underlines a number of mechanisms which are particularly important in thinking about HIV risks. The issue of mobility has already been mentioned. It is also worthwhile emphasizing once more that conflict-related mobility means that in this particular context people who joined the rebellion were most of the time out of reach and did not have access to health-related resources. Furthermore, it is interesting to consider the dates mentioned by A. He talks about the period to 93 and after 93 until the end of the conflict in terms of the availability of HIV information. This suggests that depending on the age of the combatants and the time of their participation in the rebellion, some might have entirely missed any HIV-related interventions in Burundi, including having access to condoms. As a result, the age at which a combatant becomes a part of the conflict and the duration spent with various forces are likely to be important determinants in terms of risk. This is also compounded by the way age locates people within the military hierarchy, which also had ramifications for combatants as discussed above. Here, the comment by B is informative; his claim about the fact that some were concerned about their health, albeit inadequately, since they used their eyes to assess the health of the person they were having sex with. The combination of sexual practices, the characteristics of the armed groups, and the constraints on the available HIV knowledge and resources to combatants during the conflict have implications for people who are not combatants but are impacted by the conflict in their everyday lives.

The other important part of the narrative in these interviews is the way it implicitly reflects on the nature of the conflict and how the duration of the conflict makes it difficult to have strict boundaries around who is a combatant and who is not. Here, in particular, the position of women becomes important. Their engagement with the conflict is at multiple levels. At one level they might have had husbands who might be part of the rebellion at some point. They might have been kidnapped or resorted to sex work due to the conflict. They might have joined as combatants themselves. Sometimes they are considered as a part of the armed groups by combatants themselves; sometimes they are seen as being in the background. However, what is clear is that being a non-combatant did not limit the impact of conflict on their lives. The conflict was an everyday experience for women generally.

In considering and reflecting on their experiences after the conflict the interviewees also highlight how these different aspects of their lives created complex situations for them and for others. Here the post-conflict complexity emerges as another aspect of HIV risk. They reflect on the difficulties of reintegration due to the perceptions within the community. Of course, this is also a reflection on them by the community that is based on the communities' experiences during the conflict. Difficulties in reintegrating with individual families, getting married, and dealing with multiple families emerge as important problems. For many coming back also meant that they needed to find a way of generating income. Here an important point was made by A when he talked about the need for women–wives to trust returning men–husbands. Given the nature of sexual relations, this trust clearly creates a risky situation. Trust also involved engaging with additional families for those who returned with new "bush" wives. However, they also mentioned the cases where women–wives might have had children with others while their husbands were away. The implications of this were severe for those women. Once again insecurity dominates the post-conflict context.

The discussion also highlights how the transition process from conflict to non-conflict did not engage with their needs. The process was not engaging with their experiences or the outcome of those experiences, which will impact their integration. While the process could be seen as creating a more secure environment using demilitarization, it was not dealing with the complex psychology of ex-combatants in their dealings with their communities. Part of that psychology involved thinking about HIV risks. The comment by all three interviewees about the state of shock and uncertainty which made absorbing the training they were given much harder was a common view expressed by many others. This view also implicitly questions how these transition policies are being designed. These processes are interventions to change the performativity of being a combatant and become a member of a community as an ordinary member of the society. However, the process is not straightforward, particularly considering the length of the conflict from 1993 onwards. The transformation will mean different things to different parties, depending on their position within the armed groups, how they joined, and what they did during the conflict. The switch will not be very direct even if they are on the side which becomes the government. Here the distinction between officer ranks and others is an issue which I will consider in the following chapters. The question all these points leads to is: To what extent are these processes taking into account the particular circumstances of the people? And: How far do these transition processes engage with communities and with their attitudes towards the combatants? Ultimately, the intersection between the ex-combatants and their communities will determine the outcomes of their integration. The views expressed by A are pertinent here: in most cases ex-combatants are not included in the HIV-related training and are not invited to workshops. This points out an important problem which is centrally linked to acceptance within the mainstream of society.

Most importantly perhaps, the discussion highlighted the centrality of gender attitudes in the behavior of people in the conflict. Each participant either implicitly or explicitly is talking about the implications of existing gender norms and values for governing social relations in Burundi during the conflict. This, of course, is also about gender relations in the country in general. In other words, their discussion could be seen as a reflection of gender governance in Burundi. When the interview recounts individual experiences of the conflict it is implicitly highlighting how gender positions are impacted by people's experiences and how, in particular, it created damaging conditions for women. One of the striking concepts used is voicelessness in relation to the position of women. This is perhaps the most important, since it is used when some of the interviewees talked about sexual violence. Considering that in this discussion all interviewees were men, the positionality implicit in the designation of voicelessness in the discussion is to construct women without agency. This seems to be very much linked to the lack of accessible options for women to counter and defend themselves in the face of such acts. At the same time, there is an implicit realization that the voicelessness is not a natural attribute of women but it is something related to situations produced by men. From this position women are seen without agency when facing such conditions during the conflict. While they discuss women as voiceless, it is notable that they did not talk about their agency in the same way. Although, the situations they discuss underline at a number of points their own voicelessness within the patriarchal order in which they had to function during the conflict.

The gender context one observes here is very complex. The discussion of these men's experiences suggests a challenging gender dynamic. Sexual violence was partially a way of establishing group belonging. Here there is a passing link to the argument of the creation of male fraternities through war by Lori Handrahan (2004). She argues that while men suffer tremendously in war "there is nonetheless a positive identity aspect for men to defend 'their' women and homeland" (2004: 432). This then is linked to the idea that this position of men is part of their citizenship and path for belonging in their community. After elaborating the issue by arguing that separation from the household leads to the creation of a fraternity, she concludes by asserting that "war makes the man" (2004: 433; see also Charles and Hintjens 1998). The interviews undoubtedly identify the creation of a community of rebels based on particular practices. However, a gender analysis that focuses on individual experiences, rather than considering the experiences of people according to their belonging to one or other large categorical gender positions, suggests that these communities are enforced and unstable in terms of forming male identity. The experiences of people as reported here in these communities, including the reasons why they joined the conflict, are not homogeneous. Combined with the experiences considered here, it is hard to talk about such communities of rebels as creating a positive identity for men. It seems that the process is creating a positive instrumentality for the political elite within these groups to manipulate and exploit others. Most of these manipulative tactics were based on existing gender norms and the values of what women could and could not do, stretching these to a new position in gender relations terms. These experiences had intra-gender implications for men. In the long term, sexual violence in particular seems to have, in the context of the above reported discussions, disempowered individuals while they were enforcing the patriarchal order. They managed to be part of a group at one moment in time during the conflict, as a result they were emasculated as ordinary human beings who could then not easily integrate back into their communities.

The discussion notes how gender norms are dynamically reproduced both for women and for men. The process of reproduction is linked with the regulation of their relations during the conflict. They then also point out how this reproductive process of creating and maintaining a gender order in the conflict situation is informing people's lives after the conflict. In this, women's positions in the post-conflict situation are perceived to be related to the decisions men have made during the conflict, including the decision to join the armed groups, have random sex, and take part in sexual violence. But there are also signs that women had to take decisions, such as joining the rebellion, to survive and these also had implications for their lives after the conflict too. As a result, the discussion overall points out how existing gender norms that regulate family life were challenged because of the conflict conditions. The discussion also provides a window to understand the gendered fault lines in society where various groups are made vulnerable in their everyday lives.

From this discussion, gender is emerging as an important framing issue. It is significant that interviewees identify, implicitly in most cases, gender fault lines as underwriting HIV risks during and after the conflict. The analysis they provide presents gendered relations as the structural context within which risky behavior takes place. Their views on their own behavior, as combatants among men and in relation to women, suggests that they are reflecting on what kinds of gender relations allowed these relations to develop. They are reflecting on how these relations were impacted by, for instance, mobility or being in an IDP camp. They identify particular sexual relations which they thought were risky in terms of HIV and developed in the context of the conflict. These range from sexual violence to having multiple sexual partners and issues related to condoms. There is an implicit suggestion that women were made more vulnerable in the process. They also reflect on how similar relations are produced after the conflict, creating further risk. The discussion on testing and condom use is also revealing in terms of how their gender position as men is making them resistant to engage with these issues, jeopardizing both their own lives and the lives of women they are associated with.

These interviews were a window through which we observed their concerns about the way gender relations are underwriting people's behavior across the conflict and post-conflict period. These gender boundaries regulate risky behavior. Here they raise another important question on how far the conflict impacted gender norms and how values have changed in Burundi because of the conflict. Their engagement in some of the discussion, as observed above, when they reacted to the question whether women could participate in decisions on reproductive health or whether women could demand to use condoms, demonstrates a dilemma in their own thinking about gender relations. While initially they smiled in response to these questions, it was clear that the group overall did not think these were odd questions to ask. It was just that in Burundi they did not think women had such gender agency. This was explicitly voiced as a question of women's education. However, their argument on education left their own role in making these changes possible unarticulated. Here again the gender relations underwriting this position are central for thinking about HIV risks. If men find it difficult to engage in bargaining with patriarchal norms (Connell 1996, Kandiyoti 1988) even when they can see the implications of the existing deficit in the gender relations disadvantaging women, then this is a major handicap for dealing with HIV.

Conclusion

Although this chapter is based on a single discussion, it highlighted pathways which matter for the relationship between HIV/AIDS and conflict that need to be considered. It brought out the areas that made people become concerned about HIV. On the whole, this was clearly a process for the ex-combatants that began after being exposed to the information about HIV/AIDS. They were re-evaluating their actions and experiences of the conflict. The discussion locates the debate on HIV/AIDS and conflict into personal experiences and insecurities experienced during the conflict. In other words the relationship between HIV/AIDS and conflict becomes relevant because it impacts the life of individuals and communities both during and after the conflict. The international concern for survival of the state becomes an abstract issue in this context. This is a good way to start for those who are interested in understanding how people experience the disease in conflict contexts. It allows the analysis to engage with people's experiences rather than beginning with a meta-structural concern for something called international security under which people's lives are subsumed. Furthermore, the interviews reflect on the conditions of insecurity and dislocation in their everyday lives. This is again an important aspect of the analysis here. It is imperative to consider how people lived during the conflict and why they think that there was HIV risk for them.

2 Gender relations

This chapter considers the nature of the gender norms and values that are regulating social relations in Burundi. There are several reasons to pay close attention to these norms and values. In general, gender norms and values regulate social interaction in society. Patricia O. Daley (2008) links the masculinities regulated through these norms and values to the genocidal politics observed generally in the Great Lakes region and in Burundi in particular. I agree with her that this kind of politics is about 'the erosion of respect for the sanctity of life and of the human being' (2007: 107). Gender norms and values direct individual behavior and create a way of evaluating each other's behavior in a given society. It is important to unpack how these norms and values determine the boundaries for possible ways of being to be able to see how they are then eroded by the conflict. For the purposes of this book to consider the relationship between conflict and HIV/AIDS, gender norms and values carry particular importance since, as argued by Terrell Carver (1996), these also locate the way sexual practices are deployed as power relations. Adopting such a view also challenges the way security and the HIV/AIDS framework have developed without specific reference to gender relations in conflict contexts and ignoring the importance of the gendered nature of inequalities and the way these inequalities create differentiated experiences for people (Tickner 1997).

Without gender analysis it is difficult to understand the causes of sexual violence discussed in the last chapter. Furthermore, without understanding the gendered nature of inequalities influencing people's behavior, it is difficult to uncover the mechanisms linking complex causes of sexual violence to HIV risks. Understanding these mechanisms also allows analysis to consider how conflict dynamics interact over time with gender norms and values. Here the focus is on how conflict puts existing gender norms and values under pressure and/or create opportunities for their instrumentalization in particular ways. Considering that, independent of the gender imbalances outside the conflict, rape 'was [still] a socially unacceptable act' (Daley 2007: 128), the discussion needs to understand the particularized gender norms and values and then to think about how rape had become common place in a social context which considered rape unacceptable. This question needs to be considered in a much more direct manner, rather than falling back on the existing explanations that rely on militarization or assertions of an ethnicity creating such acts (Enloe 2000: 110). Taking Daley's point about erosion of respect for sanctity seriously, one needs to consider how gender imbalances were so exacerbated that they lost some of their social control functions and were used to legitimate sexual violence. Here the issue is also about the intentional exploitation of certain gender norms during the conflict to create sexual violence (McKinnon 2006: 223). It is clear from the previous chapter that the three ex-combatants on reflection were concerned about women's position in their society. These concerns are a reaction to their own experiences, which became more devastating as they returned to their communities. The inferno section of Dante's *The Divine Comedy* ends with the lines 'and then we emerged to see the stars again' (line 139, 1998: 195). In the case of the ex-combatants this could be paraphrased as *and then we emerged to see the hell*. They found themselves reflecting on the implications of their own actions particularly in relation to women, while at the same time finding it difficult to influence a change to address the gender problem in which their own gender positions influencing their behaviors were implicated.

In the previous chapter a discussion with three ex-combatants was reported. The aim was to identify the contours of the problems that are central to our concerns on conflict and HIV/AIDS. In that discussion, gender relations emerged as central to the vulnerability structures creating HIV risks. This chapter, in order to unpack how these gender relations are shaped and operationalized, reports conversations with four women highlighting their experiences of conflict and HIV/AIDS. The women's experiences unpack and expose the foundational mechanisms of gender relations in the Burundian context. It becomes clear that these mechanisms are establishing and reproducing boundary conditions by distributing power in a differentiated manner between men and women. Men find themselves in a gender structure that maintains their power position in relation to women. Their participation in the system, which is stretched to its limits and altered during the conflict, is maintained by patriarchal dividend. In turn this patriarchal context produces power relations that have created differentiated violence for women and men (Daley 2008: 124). In the post-conflict context, men's experiences in the conflict sit unhappily in the Burundian context. This is also exacerbated for those who are not part of the political power structures and left without resources after the conflict. The gender vulnerabilities that are created in this context are also embedded in Burundian society and are influenced by the conflicts.

Interview with D

D: I live in Ngozi, I am a single child—my mother died at birth. Then I was taken in by my grandmother. When recently they found me to be HIV+, they chased me away. I don't know my father. So, with my grandmother I went to my uncle in Kayama where I was in school until the seventh grade then came back to my grandmother and when I became ill she chased me away. I was infected because I did not have a place to live. I was not able to tell my family that I was HIV+ because I looked healthy. The one who helped me went to Tanzania.

INTERVIEWER: Could you please elaborate?

D: This uncle who lived in Kayama, when the war came, he left for Tanzania. So I had to go back to my grandmother's. When I came back my grandmother's people tried to chase me away because it was not my father's place, so chased me away. This is how I became HIV+.

I do not know how it happened, I was not used to "that" [sex], I was a fine young girl. It is because my family chased me away. I had no idea how to even rent a room. I even slept outdoors, for about three months, outside like here [pointing at the grass where we were sitting]. Sometimes I was obliged to spend the night in a coffee field, and then I just got up and walked. At that point I could no longer choose boy or men. I did not know that I was getting into trouble or getting an illness. One day I thought of renting a house (after sleeping outside long time). I walked during the day like I was drunk [in a daze]. One day I got food from some organization. When I got food I rented place in the Swahili Quarter for 500 BIF per month. Now I rent this place and this whole year has been no rest, I could not sleep because I fear, I fear something could kill me.

Most of the time I preferred to live with men I accepted this because it— was hard to live outside. Some men treated me badly, other gave me some money, others give only shelter for the night—I could not push them to give me anything else. Some accepted condoms—then I thought they were healthy, other did not I thought they were HIV+ already. If I did not accept they sent me out. Because I asked to use one, if he said no and I insisted, he said "get out"—but it was too late in the night so I could not leave as I had no place to live.

INTERVIEWER: How about HIV?

D: I have been coming here [to NGO working on HIV] for nine years [at the time of the interview]. I left the seventh grade in 1993, also chased away from my grandmothers, I went to a man, I did not know the man. It was only three months. I then went out and neighbors took me in sometime, then I fell ill. I had tuberculosis and I was advised to take a test (HIV), the doctor advised. My behavior—they said was bad, it was only because I was chased away. When it happened the first time, I was healthy, only after did I become ill. Since then there has been no peace. Initially I was away for three years. I got pressure from neighbors so I came home [to the community]. I was at home a month then I fell ill and I was pushed away. I heard of HIV/AIDS first in 1993 but I didn't really know I thought I could be healed, I only knew of the severity when I came here [HIV/AIDS NGO]. Then I went for a test, with a doctor at the hospital (nine years ago) and he sent me here. I am treated well. I got advice from the doctor which I am still following, I was not so ill then. I have a very bad life now. If I did not follow advice I would probably be dead now. It is helpful to follow advice, if not you are dead. Renting a house is hard to bear.

INTERVIEWER: What was the advice?

D: Out of marriage is bad [sex], to use condoms—mostly. Even married men if you look healthy you do not want to use one. Some men accept condom, others don't. Since I rented the house I am working [sex work]. Even when I do this I really follow the advice. If the man does not accept [condom], even if he offers 10,000 BIF I cannot accept. I put my life at risk.

INTERVIEWER: Do men accept this?

They do let me go because mostly in hotels if I cry people will hear me. If I accept money without a condom I just put my life in danger. It is only for money and I like my life. In seminars women said that they ask their husbands to use condoms but don't ask others to tell him. Then I say—tell your husbands he must accept. If not, you do not accept. I have a friend whose husband does not listen. I say "go away then" but she refuses. She is now ill so it is hard to abandon. Other women are in similar position. My friends from Marangaro commune, they are separated once women became healthy. They have a child together so they went together, then she got ill—I advised her to leave again. But she wanted to raise the child together. I asked the doctor to give her this advice but she would not listen. I advised her to go out of the rented house and get another one. They were not married they lived together. If they live together she will get pregnant again. She is too weak and a child would make her worse.

If a man came to me and said 'let's live together' I know he will not accept regulations [use of condom]. He would only accept it for a few days and that will put me into trouble. So, I prefer to live alone, if I wanted I could have sex with condoms and then go home. If we are married, he can only accept for a few days and then I would be in trouble. Then if you insist, he will kick you out, then you are on your own again, so why even start?

Many men in towns do not accept condoms, in rural area it is different. Rural men would discuss and won't go with other women. In towns if a woman insists (to use a condom) he could go find another woman. Man in rural areas, if they chase their wives, everyone will know, and follow the woman, the man could be laughed at. In towns they say "if you refuse there are many women looking for men so, be careful, tomorrow you could be out."

INTERVIEWER: Can't that also happen in rural areas?

D: If the couple is HIV+ and the man chases the women out people would laugh. Here in town, men could know he is HIV+ but still live with two or three wives. For instance in the Swahili Quarter, there is a Congolese man with three wives—two HIV+ and the third HIV- (one Rwandese, one Tutsi Burundian, and one Congolese). All live in the same compound. Many people know their status but what is dangerous is that they test in far away places and do not reveal their status and keep infecting.

It is hard to negotiate [family planning]. You see many healthy children but many who are not. May be they become ill and die and don't have the chance to even raise the child. Also, when you are HIV+ people die because of malaria. It is hard when you are pregnant and HIV+ with malaria.

Interview with E

E: My family chased me away; I don't live with them since July 2007. After I gave birth they chased me. I came to live here [Gitega], I told them [women she is sharing the house with] about my problems and they accepted me here. Came here in this house, my mother does not want me to live here [found out later that her mother wanted her at home but her brothers did not]. I went to live in another house in the compound. Saturday I went and asked for forgiveness, my mother accepted but my two brothers refused. Then I told them here that my family had refused me and they accepted me here. The problem is because the father of the child died in July. With my husband we lived both at home, his home, near Songa, near the fuel tanks [large government stocks]. Then he died and we were not officially married, his family pushed me away. I live with the woman who helped me, without her I would be on the streets with no food. I do not have any money to go and do business like others. I have relatives in Bujumbura but no one will help me. I still wait for forgiveness. I am thankful to God for everything. Difficult, very difficult when your family don't want to help you and chase you away. You have no life.

INTERVIEWER: You were not officially married? …

E: The pregnancy was not planned, it was while I was at the school, we had not planned to get married. My relations were not bad with my mother-in-law with the father-in-law not good. My husband told me that I was too young to properly manage a house so said go home. They only wanted to keep the child. I cannot give them my child, he is too young, he needs me, he is nearly three now.

INTERVIEWER: You said your brothers refused forgiveness, could you please elaborate?

E: One of them said 'go back to your place [husband's] we don't want to see you pregnant'. It was very difficult. My mother tried to convince him, she tried to find people to help but my brothers refused. One is a driver if he sees me on the street he will kill me with his car. I cannot go home I know they are there. The other one has a taxi moto he too is very hard with me. Those in the neighborhood are fine with me, I am only afraid of my brothers. One brother is officially married and the other is kind of engaged, bride-price [dowry] is done. The older one says don't go to bed before marriage, his wife gave birth two months after they married.

INTERVIEWER: Is this about land?

E: Yes, because all my sisters and my father are dead there is no other person of authority. My elder sister was married now a widow with two kids. They say go to your husband's family to raise my son, because he is a boy. They said 'we don't want to see a boy here'. So they don't forgive me. It is very unjust, it happens to many young women [being pregnant] I make them [the family] feel very ashamed because I came back to give birth and that brings bad luck, I am a 'bad girl;', my husband died, I was treated unjustly.

My husband was ill, he got sick on July 3rd and on July 8th he was dead. At the time of death his family was negative. They did not want to give me land, they only wanted the child and I will give him when he is older. I had good relations with his family

INTERVIEWER: What do you do?

E: I have no job. Health services are free for my son. I wish for a job but it is not possible. For a job I would like a small capital, to have money for food.

INTERVIEWER: How do you stay here?

E: I knew her [landlady] from before, I used come here when I was a student. She has a good heart and accepted me here she said 'if I have food I will share it with you'. The woman does not ask me for rent, sometimes my brother or sister from Bujumbura send money to help. It is very difficult here but there is no way to avoid this.

The pattern of family break down that is observed in both women's discussions is common among most of our interviewees. The striking statement common in most of these discussions has been the statement that *I don't have a family*, which is followed by the statement that they live or have mothers or matrilineal relations. These unpack what is considered to be family that matters for women to survive in their communities. A close look at these statements allows the analysis to engage with the foundational gender framework in Burundi. The interviews indicate that men either as a father or as a husband, or if the father/husband is dead or has left, a male relative is central for the livelihoods of women. In other words, marriage and the family it forms reproduce gender relations. The Burundian family is both patriarchal and patrilocal. In a traditional setting, men are defined as the stable, core, central, and identity-founding part of the "family," while women are defined as the unstable, peripheral, and relational-(ex)changing part of the family: women are what a family can get from outside, and can concede without important loss. This has important consequences, in terms of women's vulnerabilities and men's responsibilities (and advantages) attached to their respective roles.

The social position of women is determined by her male network through her father and husband. However, as a general attitude women's social and legal position is considered to be ambiguous: women are either coming from other families when men marry, or as sisters and daughters who will join other families. In the former husband's family they will treat a woman in relation to her husband's position in his own family. This will be particularly important when the husband becomes absent and the wife needs to live with his family. In the latter case absence of a father matters a lot as the sister becomes subject to her brothers' attitudes towards her. Also, this gender situation, in which power is distributed unequally, is unequally maintained and exacerbated for women through the legal mechanisms of property ownership. Women do not own property, which would include land, animals, and houses, and also they lack the right to inherit property. Here as it is clear from the extracts above male relatives also like to maintain control over their economic resources and do not want to share these with their sisters or sisters-in-law. They expect each to be supported: in the case of a sister by their husband's family and in the case of a sister-in-law they are expected to rely on their own father's family, as in the absence of a husband wives do not have the familial link with their in-laws.

This gender system undoubtedly creates a generalized vulnerability for women independent of the conflict context. A woman's position in a community is a function of her male network. In the idea of the family, men are the stable part of the social structure. Women could navigate this system depending on their male network, particularly in relation to their paternal links. In the absence of powerful men supporting women who are related, to them the system will create severe vulnerabilities for those women. It is clear that the system is vulnerable in the conflict due to the absorption of men into various armed groups over extended periods of time. Such change has meant that women have lost many important links in their male networks that they need to be able to pressurize the system.

Also important, as Peter Uvin (2009: 125) emphasizes, is marriage. It remains an important social structure through which both men and women achieve adulthood. Gender structures are reproduced and affirmed through the form of family that is created in this process. In most of the interviews when a person talks about marriage it is traditional marriage. This highlights another important gendered process that maintains and at the time of conflict creates further vulnerabilities for women. Formal legally registered and binding marriage is rare. It is important to unpack this process to understand why this process creates vulnerabilities.

Legally binding marriage is only performed before government authorities in commune offices. The traditional marriage is in place after the performance of certain steps: first, contact needs to happen between two families through arrangement by marriage brokers who are known to have a positive image in the community; then the payment of the bride-price takes place. Then the marriage ceremony takes place as public and private activities. The public marriage ceremony includes a convoy for the bride, which is made up of chanting young women and men accompanying the bride to her future husband's home. The private marriage ceremony includes practices performed in the house of the groom by both the young man and the young bride. The highly symbolic moment, traditionally said to be the very moment of marriage, is when the groom snatches the bride's clothes off her, and gives her new clothes that he has bought for her. This is a transformative moment, a ritual, where the woman achieves a new status by the removal of her clothes provided by her father and by wearing the clothes bought by her husband she acquires a new family and home. The old clothes are sent back with an aunt who might have been part of the wedding convoy. Once this process is completed, the couple is considered to be married.

In this traditional context marriage is of course binding in its own way. Once it is performed and the bride-price is paid, the husband is expected to recognize children born out of the marriage, look after his wife, and provide shelter for her. The wife is entitled to cultivate her husband's land even when he is absent for a period. The husband is responsible for the protection of his wife. As Uvin argues, traditionally:

> for the first two years or so after the marriage, the family of the groom supports the new couple in various ways, including by preparing their meals. This ends with a ceremony in which young family becomes independent. At this point, the husband acquires full financial and social responsibility for his wife and children.
>
> (Uvin 2009: 125)

If the husband is going to be absent for a period he traditionally asks his male relatives, such as his father, brothers, or uncles, to perform these roles and look after his *home*. This particular situation is known to create vulnerabilities for the wife. The marriage is binding for women too. They cannot continue to live in their parents' house and land. A woman has to go to her husband's house and work on his land. Also, she needs to stay at home while the husband could be away at the market or visiting others.

The question of how binding this marriage is is an important one. It seems that for a man, it is binding when he accepts it. It is not so binding when he wants to divorce his wife. In this traditional marriage a wife cannot, by her own, challenge her husband or his relatives. If she manages to do so it usually indicates that she has a strong male network including her father, brothers, or uncles which is respected by her husband's family. Here the power could be related to wealth, socio-political connections, or as having more family members than the husband's family. A woman could not alone invoke the bride-price in order to enforce a marriage. The husband, on the other hand, uses the bride-price to his advantage—he could say that I paid the price because I wanted you. But, he could argue and create reasons, if he wishes to do so, why he does not want to be married anymore. This could include reasons such as claims that the woman "doesn't obey me," "does not respect me," "does not cook well," "comes late at home," or "even being drunk." These are accepted reasons used in many divorces by the *bashingantahe* to dismiss a woman.

Here, it is important to note that the gender power imbalance in family life is a problem. It is maintained and reproduced by the precarious marriage arrangements that make women subservient in the relationship. The situation discussed, however, also shows that there are avenues open to women to influence this relationship as long as her male network is supportive. This gender imbalance is based on both the enforcement and ability to enforce through such networks the implications of the bride-price and the recognition of the marriage processes performed. Given what is considered to be a relevant indicator of power, not all women who enter such marriages are able to enforce their views in the relationship.

Furthermore, many men and women live together, cohabit, and when a woman begins living in a man's accommodation they often declare that they are married. This is because the traditional marriage process is beyond many people's and their families' means. Therefore, many marriages do not involve a bride-price. The resulting process means that the couple is looked after by the husband's family. Therefore, even the basic responsibility, independent of the weakness identified above, created by the bride-price is not applicable in many cases. In more informal marriages the enforceability of marriage becomes purely a function of men's willingness to remain in that relationship. In this, women are highly vulnerable, as decisions are taken by men. In addition, most social and legal rules support men in their socio-political position, for example, all assets are owned by men. Even the identity of belonging to a group, like family, and its ascendance are traced solely along male members thus further weakening women's socio-political position. In this environment, men are relied upon to protect, support, and speak for their wives, sisters, and mothers.

Early on, until the 1980s the government tolerated traditional marriages and accepted to legalize them. However, the government at present tends only to recognize legal marriage. In the 1980s, the government also declared the 'bride-price' illegal. This, however, has not led to the wide acceptance and compliance with legal marriage. One of the reasons for this is the financial difficulties, identified by Uvin (2009: 128), for men to perform traditional requirements of marriage. Another problem is related to the gender imbalances in decision-making power, that women cannot force men to have legal marriages. The informal marriage process is by and large considered normal, and as observed in many interviews allows women to have some male support. However, as Uvin points out "the cost of it [informal marriage] is largely borne by women. Indeed, such arrangements put her at risk" (2009: 128). As a result there is a complex problem whereby many people would argue that they have been married while the commune might not recognize this claim. The claimant needs to prove that they have been married according to the legal documentation to be able to get formal support in her cause. At present there are NGOs running programs to help couples register their marriage in the commune, thus legalizing it. These programs aim to protect women and children given that traditional marriage is not secure.

The traditional gender governance distributing differentiated power in society by controlling differentiated access to socio-political and economic resources also has a multidimensional inter-generational impact. It is clear that children located in the context of traditional marriage will have unpredictable family lives that depend very much on their sex on the one hand and the support their mothers have in the broader male networks on the other. In this family context in the absence of the husband, both girl and boy children might be kept by the husband's family. However, in practice this happens more often with the sons, with the mother and the daughters being sent away or back to the mother's family if they accept. Also depending on the relationship between the mother and her in-laws she might be allowed to stay while looking after the children. These processes are not random choices but linked to the gender governance emerging from the analysis above. Children also function as a part of this process with traditionally recognized entitlements that are also gender specific. While a woman after her husband's death could be sent away, a son would still maintain his claim over his father's property. Also, the example reported in E's case above, having a son, even from someone else, increases her claims towards her own family too. However, the difficulty in most of these circumstances is the conditions under which women can enforce either of these entitlements. Here for the enforceability to have access to resources, legally recognized marriage becomes an important tool. At the same time, these resource implications in the context of a declining resource base in the country from the conflict creates one of the reasons why men resist legally binding marriage. The circumstances for girls are also precarious, depending on their mother's ability to provide for them. This creates a vicious circle which is the outcome of gender governance that is hard to break for a young girl. As a result, she might find herself destitute without any resources.

Interview with F

F: I was divorced this January (2007). He has another life now. When married, we were not legally married. He was a rebel fighter and had no time for legal marriage. So after he came from the bush we got married [not in the commune]. I could not convince him to go to the commune. The other woman, they were together in the bush, I did not know. They are both in the police now. After the bush the other woman was in Bujumbura. When we separated he went to Bujumbura to find her now they are both in Bujumbura. The other woman knows both came to see when I had the baby; he does not help with the baby. The child is legally recognized at the commune but there is no other help.

I see HIV+, I am HIV+. I lived with my husband but we are separated and now he has a second wife. When I was tested and found out I was HIV + he divorced me and got a second wife. Since then I had a bad life. I have no parents I rent a house. I decided to look for a living but because I was HIV + it is hard to find work. I have no food, no soap I wish I had a small capital or job to abandon this work. Men promise money, do things to you, and not pay you and even beat you up. You could say no the man "I am HIV+" and he could say "so what I came from somewhere you could give it to me, we could get other diseases." Now you see people are dying men sometimes accepts condom.

INTERVIEWER: Tell us about your background?

F: I am from Ngozi, I was born here. I have no family, I live with my mother, my brother and father were killed in Rwanda. My father went to work in business and my brother joined RPF [Rwandan Patriotic Front]. My mother she does not do anything—only sells little charcoal. I have no job, I only sell tomatoes in the market but sometimes I only get 1000 BIF or keep the tomatoes too long and they rot, it is a very small capital. I only had 5000 BIF capital and now only have 3000 and tomatoes are expensive, a bucket is 8000 BIF. People come to the market buy the whole basket, in order to sell now I go to Kayanza. I also had a case of Primus [beer] however they recently stole the full case during the night they broke in and stole the beer and the cloths. I live in bad conditions; I am not sure how I can get money.

INTERVIEWER: Do men approach you when you are selling beer?

F: I am never bothered because there are others [sex workers]. There are no men coming to me (at home) because I live with my mother.

INTERVIEWER: How do you meet men if they come to you?

F: I ask for another room from friends. When this happens I share the money with the other woman whose room it is. Beforehand I had capital I did not have to work this way [sex work] now there are bad conditions I need to do it.

INTERVIEWER: How frequently do you have work?

F: Some women who have many go to hotels. I only have those who are not rich may be could only pay 1000–2000 BIF. Those women in the hotels have clients often because they are in hotels. Those men have lots of money. In the compound I sold beer men came for beer and asked me to show them a woman and then I called someone. There were many men like this. They came usually at the end of the month after they were paid. Many who come to the hotel have money, even Mzungu [foreigner] like you, they pay 5,000–10,000 BIF not like in the home. Many come from Bujumbura, also people who come for work here, they ask guards to find someone for them. Sometimes they are civil servants, independent business men-Mzungus you see them in the hotels.

INTERVIEWER: Why did you go testing and how was it?

F: I was pregnant in December and I tested after. I went before pregnancy. I saw my husband taking medication but he was not ill. I thought that was strange. So I asked friends and they said those who take medications all the time may be HIV+, especially if it is Backtrim, so I went for a test. I found out I was HIV+ I came and told him, he became angry. At that point I said "well you take medication" (to imply that he might be HIV+) and he said that he takes it because he is tired. We argued blaming each other for the infection then we split.

INTERVIEWER: Did you receive PMCT [prevention of mother-to-child transmission]?

F: Yes I took the medicine to protect the child. I took advice and I will only breastfeed until six months. If there is no help though, it is hard to find money if I stop breastfeeding because I don't have enough milk.

INTERVIEWER: How do people treat you?

F: Some avoid me because I am HIV+ some discriminate if you ask for something they refuse to share with you. My mother has problems we live together but she has eye problems needs soap. I cannot ask for soap she says "go to the husband." The neighbors don't treat me badly. I am not generally treated badly my mother is poor, I need to pay for the rent that's the problem.

INTERVIEWER: Have you sought assistance to get your husband to help with the baby?)

F: I am thinking about it, I heard the police people will soon be demobilized, may be I do not have the means. I just raise the child. The baby is a girl. Once she is grown may be she will be his child. I know where he lives, Muhanga commune. He has brothers and his mother. His brother is rich business men. When I go and say the child is ill. They could give money to help. The husband never, they will never accept her.

Interview with G

The following extract is from an interview with a woman who was supporting herself as a sex-worker in Ngozi Town. At the time of the interview she was 20 and had a seven-year-old child. At the beginning she thought she and the father of the child had planned the child as he rented a house for them to live together. However, immediately after the birth, she realized that he was having relations with many other women. She believes that she has HIV because of him. After she learned her HIV status he refused to support them (her and her child) and treated her badly. She left home to live with her mother. He married another woman.

G: There are groups talking about HIV/AIDS, but only to women. They taught us in seminars how to live, how to behave (sexually), how to protect us ourselves, and distributed condoms at the end. They teach us that one has to make efforts to live well and protect yourself, especially if you are HIV+—that you need to use condom all the time, even when you make a living from sex.

INTERVIEWER: Is there a discrimination against PLWHA?

G: Some people discriminate against you others not because in the place where we live, most neighbors are HIV+ so there is no discrimination. In other neighborhoods if they know you are HIV+ they will most likely to discriminate against you.

INTERVIEWER: How are community relations?

G: Because we go on the street, we need to look for food for our children when one receives food, they don't share (there is a sort of competition, there is no solidarity, no community). In the neighborhood it is hard, because neighbors' activities are the same as your [sex work] she might have had someone that night so you could not ask them for food.

NGO [local branch of an Africa-wide NGO network] helps with me and my child. Before they gave food but now they do not [under new World Food Program guidelines only those on ARVs are given food aid]—they only give medication. Some take Bactrim (an antibiotic) and others ARVs, it is the doctor who decides. I take Backtrim. Sometimes I stop it makes me hungry—it's hard. Few men respect women, few respect the voice of women.

INTERVIEWER: Why?

G: Men do not respect women, some are friendly and nice. However some are violent after sex they beat you up and don't pay. Some could be, God willing, kind. They could come and talk about HIV, condoms, and protection. Men are willing to use condoms. But not all of them. You could give the man a condom and he just wears it, then you could use the female condom and sometimes he does not even know. I try to this all the time if he refuses the condom. If the man refuses the condom, some could accept the female condom. Some refuses both so you need to be smart—they showed us how to put the female condom well so that it is hidden, so he does not know. We always use the condom, we have been taught, if he does not accept, I prefer to say no and go hungry.

G: I cannot count them [men] there are many, many, many—some are not married, some are, those ones try and hide themselves. Some are employed— many are drivers. It is not the men often looking for us, we have to go and find, we find them—we go where they are, to bars. We go out to be seen. We work, of course, everyday, if not, how do we have a life?

Authorities respect us but when it is late they [police] beat us—this still happens now. When you are in bars and they want to close, some girls say "I will not go home without at least 1,000 BFS [approximately US$1 at the time]" so go and wander on the streets. Sometimes you are somewhere [on the street] and they [police] keep you there [on the street]—because you are out too late (in Burundian culture no 'good' woman stays out late). They are enforcing an unofficial curfew, making us walk with them or sit with them as one type of punishment, then as another type of punishment insist that you sleep together, and you accept for your safety. They [police] even take your money, rape and/or beat you.

INTERVIEWER: So you have family who could help?

G: I have no family [tears streaming down] I have a mother who is very poor. It [life] is hard.

I have asked for help to get out of this bad life, asked for credit, sometimes I am hungry all day and into the night. But up to now there is no help. We really want help, we did not choose this, it is poverty forcing us. We need help, I have only one mother, who is poor, no father, brother, or sisters, no land, no house—I have to rent. I still talk to my mother, but I am poor. I wish, because I have no family, that I could have a small capital, I would buy some peanuts and sell them on the street. Sometimes I go three days without eating.

There is no doubt that the norms and values underpinning the gender governance in Burundi were absolutely making women vulnerable before the conflict. As this governance mechanism is the common background to the way the society functions, the inequalities it underwrites "become invisible and accepted as the norm" (Handrahan 2004: 430). The gender governance regulates the resource relations that are central for the survival and the socio-political participation in the decision-making processes that determine women's livelihoods. This governance mechanism concentrates power and resources within male-dominant networks. By its assignment of resources and power to the male networks it engenders compliance within the male network and reproduces the system. This is an extreme case of durable inequality (Tilly 1999). Gender governance of this kind also creates complications and competition for resources among women. In some cases, the power imbalances are forcing mothers to let their daughters go. In other circumstances there are chains of relations around one man with a succession of wives brought into a relationship. In this latter case there are further important issues. One is how men are able to manipulate their marriage obligations and how fast they can get in and out of the traditional arrangements. Another is how changing circumstances, depending on men's attitudes towards marriage, make women more acquiescent within the marriage. This allows men to maintain their power position in the marriage. Lastly, if husbands have relations with other women and/or set up a new home with other women, many wives find themselves with diminishing resources available for their wellbeing and survival. Women within this gender governance find themselves exposed to unexpected socio-economic compromises such as resorting to sex-work, including temporary transactional sex, to survive. Gender governance here is creating further vulnerabilities outside of marriage. A woman's vulnerability in marriage or in a family is also reproduced as a result of this governance. Since a woman's position in society is mediated by her position in the family, for women who find themselves outside the family structures and networks, their lives become much harder.

G's comments highlight the framework within which women need to function if they are not part of a family network mediated by their marriage. If a woman is outside the marriage it means she needs to deal with men and their advances on her own. They cannot rely on any protection, even if they resort to engaging with the police as indicated by G. Ironically, by being outside marriage, women seemed to have moved out of basic social mechanisms limiting people to take advantage of them or abuse them. The position of being open to this kind of abuse is the function of gender leverage provided to men. Gender governance seems to create damaging outcomes for women at each level. In some ways gender governance has constructed social relations in such a way that women in public become even more vulnerable to the opportunistic relations men establish.

In relation to HIV/AIDS this is of course a very dramatic problem as most of the discussions reported here indicate one of the main problems is to negotiate condom use. Women don't seem to have any leverage to influence men's behavior. For instance, even if they find someone to marry, it becomes difficult for them to negotiate formal registration. This then for them creates an unstable process of establishing a family, as shown in the discussion with D. The family life that is discussed by F in this regard also shows that, for instance, diagnosis with HIV led her husband to leave her and she had to find alternative ways to support herself and her child, creating further vulnerabilities for both of them. The survival mechanisms that are available to women lead to a cycle where at each step women become more disadvantaged as a result of the previous actions they have taken to survive.

The existence of this gender governance in society does not mean that everyone agrees with its boundaries. The discussion in the previous chapter shows that even some male ex-combatants have questions in their minds about gender relations. In other words, some agree and some comply with these gender norms and values. There is a diversity of views among both women and men. If this diversity exists then the question is: What is it that allows women from different age groups and backgrounds to be treated in this manner? So far the discussion has highlighted the way socio-economic and legal resources are distributed in an unequal manner, creating a gender imbalance among women and men at the expense of the former. It is also clear that in time this gender governance has inculcated particular attitudes and led certain behaviors to develop. Here the women's behavior is also important. While they find men's approach to them at times abusive, they also find it difficult to change this situation. An important explanation, given by many we interviewed, involves looking at the way women are instructed in their gender roles within families and communities. Many point out that women are supposed to be socially passive, and this behavior is developed in the family through an imposed shyness. In reflecting on his research on Burundi, Uvin points out that "for young women, the stream of values of obedience, moral behavior, and politeness and respectfulness comes first. The proportion of answers centering on "obedience" and "morality" are three times higher for women than for men; "politeness and respectfulness score six times higher' (Uvin 2009: 135). As a part of this world women are expected *not* to talk about sex, or participate in any discussion of, for instance, how many children they want to have or whether to use condoms or not. According to a female gender specialist from Bujumbura:

> Everything is linked to gender. We need to break the taboo. Burundian girl does not say NO. She just has a shy gesture: she hides her face. And men will just say: if she does this it means she agrees. We need to talk openly of all these things so we can fight effectively against injustice, and achieve real empowerment. On sexual issues, it's all the same for women. Taboo is for all women. A woman cannot say to a man: 'I want you'. It is difficult for women to talk about sexuality, even if the woman has an important place in the family. When a woman is a minister, something

changes. The change is about an individual capacity that is enforced. But culture is important: you will see some women mocking other women's efforts. Or women will advise other women to accept the wrong situation, by saying: "Ni ko zubakwa"—this is how household is built. The fact that the woman cannot communicate about sex caused sometimes couples to break apart. You know, when things are not well in bed, things are bad everywhere.

This is but one part of their apparent shyness in public. "Public" should be considered broadly here. When a family has visitors, for instance, one can observe this shyness both in relation to the wife of the host and their daughters. Neither wife nor daughter would participate in the discussion or express their views. When they are approaching the guest they do speak but only in whispering tones so not to interfere with the ongoing chatter. This is concrete and physical voicelessness. What is observed here is the intergenerational instruction on behavior whereby young girls learn by observing older women and their relationships with their father as well as other men. This shyness means that if they are alone in public without the family, men can instrumentalize this gender trait, as reported above by G. Her discussion of the way both she and other women who are doing sex work are treated by police is a reflection of this shyness. If she is stopped by a powerful man, here the police, she consents to be held without much explanation. This tacit acknowledgment of the power of men is a well-established situation. Gradually she agrees to things as led by men. She cannot in most cases say "OK enough is enough I am going home" before the policeman agrees to let her go.

The implications of this particular position for women were also highlighted by a Burundian gender and HIV/AIDS specialist who was at the time of the interview working for an international organization:

Community knows HIV is a big health and development problem. They wish they know how to deal with it. We had an Art competition and 1200 people across the country participated we saw in what they produced that they know the problem. If you look at what they have done, in fact there is a sort of culture, there is a line they don't want to cross, sexuality. Perception of sex determines their vulnerability. Sex in Burundian context is male privilege. It is who asks, decides how to have sex, where and when. It is the male who is the actor of the sexual act, the female is the recipient. She is not to object, female knows that she is there for the pleasure of the men, it is her duty. Man has to pay dowry (and sex is covered in it). It is because he has paid she must and should have sex with her man. She cannot contradict her husband it is not accepted. She would not consider baby her own but husbands family. We need to change men and then things change in the family. If women change and men remain the same there will be conflict. Women are empowered but cannot change things. For instance, the use of radio is the best channel for knowledge as people cannot read. If people have enough radios it would be really good. But, when you have a radio at home it's the possession of man. He controls the radio. He has good reasons to turn it off [as there are many gender-related programs on it]. Having batteries is another issue. He says that "do you buy them? I buy them I decide." He turns it on when he wants as he wants to save the batteries. If he is not there she still cannot use it as she cannot buy batteries. Even if you develop a program you really don't know whether they hear it.

The imbalance among genders in relation to sexual behavior is also highlighted by another social worker who was engaged in HIV and health training for women:

I was in a training [for a national NGO] group in discussion and I asked: "Who ever touched husband's sex [penis]?" No one had tried. Then I told them to try and tell me next time. Later, women told me: "We did it, it's nice. You are wonderful. It's good."

Women's presumed gender position is initiating imposition of a particular kind of behavior as the normal way of being. This behavior once learned at a young age becomes habitual for a lifetime. The process allows patriarchal control over women to be maintained and the way they have access to social and economic resources. In other words, it is about regulating women's public and private life by controlling their voices. The interview extracts above highlight the multiple levels of women's voicelessness. This is also related to the intra-gender process according to different ages and status of women. Here the radio example is instructive in terms of the bind women find themselves in. The fact that talking about sex is a male domain creates an immediate problem for women's lives. Women are aware of their own needs; the problem here is instead how to bring these needs as objects of open discussion, without being further penalized for doing so. The point is about the constant reproduction of unequal power relations from the private to the public spheres. In some ways, the distinction is not relevant for the women's position as they are made voiceless in private as a way of controlling their behavior in public. This situation results in a further problem of audibility. Since women are not expected to speak; when they do speak it is not clear who will listen in this context. Furthermore, the interviews reported in this chapter show how vulnerabilities are created through being voiceless. This then leads to a series of socio-economic handicaps for women, while reproducing gender governance. The system is creating vulnerabilities for HIV and has other health implications. It creates a problem for instance for talking about HIV. While at the same time, the situation is allowing men more space to engage in sexual relations. This is clearly an important structural issue that creates conditions for the spread of HIV.

Conclusion

This chapter has highlighted the mechanism of gender governance that reg-ulates people's lives in Burundi. This was done by concentrating on the experiences of four women whose lives demonstrated gender problems experienced by many others we interviewed. The mechanisms identified by these women include socio-economic and legal processes that are deployed in particular ways to allow men to have more control in society, thus creating a patriarchal context. Furthermore, it is clear that this order is reproduced in women's and men's lives through the normalization of particular behaviors, such as the silence women observe in their dealings with men in public. The submissiveness this entails makes their needs appear insignificant. Their apparent support embodied in their silence enforces unwilling compliance to men's status. These regulatory attitudes allow women to be controlled and easily exposed to abuse, particularly at times of conflict.

The conflict has no doubt changed a number of dynamics in the society that underlined these social relations. The interview with D above shows the instability sparked by the conflict that was experienced by a young woman. Her experi-ence also shows the gendered implications of the changes in social relations it has brought about. As pointed out above women traditionally stay at home and do not stay out after dark in rural areas. In those circumstances men's mobility was still a way for these women to be impacted by HIV/AIDS. With the conflict, large numbers of women were left without their husbands and, both as a result of this and violence, were pushed out of villages and homes. They were forced to be mobile, travelling either across the country or into IDP camps.

In Burundi this process of being alone, being highly mobile, and facing a break from the traditional positions did not result in greater empowerment (Rehn and Johnson-Sirleaf 2002; Handrahan 2004: 435–36; Fuest 2008: 209; Pankhurst 2008: 22–23). On the contrary, women's lives became more pre-carious. Violence against women not only happened across the political or ethnic divides but it was a common intra-community and intra-ethnic occur-rence. The gender governance that was unpacked in this chapter here high-lights the vulnerability structures that are part of society, both before and during the conflict. It is not that women cannot decide about issues impacting their lives, but it is more about how gender governance creates mechanisms allowing patriarchal norms to shape their decision-making processes. HIV risks are linked to the various ways vulnerabilities are experienced by people under circumstances determined by their social and economic positions. The relationship between conflict and HIV should be understood as a function of how these structural vulnerabilities are put under stress. The analysis needs to engage with the ways these stresses exacerbate existing gender imbalances and create new vulnerabilities. The implications of these conflict-related changes are important for understanding people's needs after the conflict. The key to this is to recognize that the link between conflict and HIV/AIDS is a relationship that acts in people's everyday lives.

3 Gender relations in the conflict

This chapter focuses on the way the long conflict in Burundi impacted gender relations. It is this relationship that is important for understanding the possible links between HIV and the conflict. In Burundi, living conditions changed due to the high mobility of the armed groups, including the regular army, and mobilization, which was stretched out over long period from 1993 onwards. The changing circumstances and constant mobility of people due to the conflict across the country put pressures on gender relations. Gender relations were gradually put under stress as greater numbers of men joined the rebellion or the military to fight. Women were made homeless, were exposed to violence, were raped, and endured being taken into the rebellion to perform various roles that exacerbated women's gender vulnerabilities and created new ones. These experiences intensified traditional gender norms leading to women's vulnerabilities. They also indicate a significant change in gender relations when the traditional mechanism of control eroded. However, this situation does not fit what is described as a "break down" of "patriarchal structures, and women gain as an unintended consequences, freedom, responsibility and worth" (Handrahan 2004: 436). While traditional gender mechanisms were stretched to their limits, norms and values underwriting these structures, such as expected behavior types in public, were instrumentalized to such an extent that women become severely vulnerable. The critical issue is about the way the changing social context in a conflict situation deploys traditional gender tropes to instrumentalize women and their labor. This does not show the disappearance of the patriarchy. Rather it indicates a hyper-patriarchal reconfiguration whereby the existing patriarchal structures identified with marriage and family are replaced by the structures of arms and camps as the regulatory structural basis for gender relations. The following interview material, for instance, highlights how younger women without patrilineal protection became destitute. While the absence of patrilineal protection made women vulnerable, the general patriarchal gender norms facilitated men's exploitation of these vulnerabilities during the conflict. In other words, the analysis of experiences indicates the instrumentalization of the rationale of existing gender norms to justify and legitimate practices that materialized in the context of the conflict. It is at this juncture that the questions about HIV risks also

emerge. However, before looking at the experiences and considering the changing gender vulnerabilities during the conflict I would like to provide a short
outline of the conflict dynamics. This adds relevant background information.

The sources of conflict date from the early years of post-independence
Burundi. The events of the 1972 "Hutu rebellion" were important for creating
a large number of displaced people. The suppression of the Hutu population
and violence against the local Hutu elite and their supporters by the government
was severe. According to René Lemarchand, 'thirty-five years ago Burundi
was the scene of a horrific bloodletting when from late April to September
1972 anywhere between 200,000 to 300,000 Hutu were massacred by a Tutsi-
dominated army. When the slaughter stopped, most of the educated adult
Hutu males were either dead or in exile" (Lemarchand 2009: 129). She also
states that between 1972 and 1973 "an estimated 200,000 Burundians, mainly
Hutu, fled the country (Daley 2008: 69). Nigel Watt argues that 'the venom
created in 1972 is the background to all the subsequent history of the country" (2008: 34). While the ethnic divide can be observed in these conflicts, it is
also important to point out that the intra-ethnic divide is sometimes related
to regional differences and that this is one of the characteristics of Burundian
politics (Watt 2008: 106). In the 1972 events, although the government targeted the Hutu it is not clear how far local Hutu supported a rebellion that
was motivated by refugee communities from outside the country. In the same way,
the government's response was also seen as a way of dealing with Tutsi who did
not agree with the government. One of the main characteristics of the conflict
in Burundi, the movement of displaced people across the country and out of
the country because of violence, was also already established by this period.

The conflict following 1993 can be seen as a conflict between the government and multiple small armed groups. The national army was deployed to
deal with the opposition while the national army forced the Hutu population
to be relocated into camps in order to stop their assumed help and support
for the rebel groups. Tutsi were also displaced by the movement of rebel
groups. In their report entitled *Burundi: Breaking the Deadlock,* published in
May 2001, the International Crisis Group states that:

> life expectancy at birth, which was 44 years in 1970, had increased by
> almost ten years in 1992, but subsequently dropped to 42 years in 1997.
> In 1998, 60 percent of the rural population and 67 percent of the urban
> population was living below the poverty level, compared to 25 and 35
> percent, respectively in 1992.

> (ICG 2001: 11)

They also look at the impact of the conflict on people's movement within and
outside the country and stated that:

> in February 2001, a total of 390,000 people from Burundi were registered
> refugees by the UNHCR, of whom 370,000 were in Tanzania alone.

During the same period, over 380,000 Burundians were displaced inside the country in 210 reported sites. Over 120,000 displaced people have not returned to those sites or their homes since July 2000, making the total number of displaced people about 500,000 people.

(ICG 2001: 11)

Furthermore, new fighting in the early months of 2001 around Bujumbura created another displacement for an additional "54,000 people" (Ibid.). At the time of publication of this report in May 2001, most of these people were still displaced and unwilling to return to their homes. It is also important to emphasize the fact that both the military and other armed groups were constantly moving across the country. It is said that the rebel groups were moving in to fight with the military around Gishubi, Mutaho, Nyarusange, Bukirasazi communes in Gitega province, and in the regions of Ruyigi, Rutana, and Cankuzo leading into Kibira. The exact routes they followed to reach their destination both from their camps in the country and after they entered the country from Tanzania are still considered to be sensitive information. One of the female ex-combatant interviewees did, however, talk openly about it: "About the hypothetical passage—it is not only hypothetical, it is indeed a passage and it caused loss of life, the groups caused damage." When juxtaposed with the displaced people, the movement of military and other armed groups created an environment which made women, in particular, very vulnerable. Also, central here is the time component of the conflict. Its prolonged nature is another important characteristic of the conflict. Gradually, women were becoming more and more impoverished and exposed. The stress put on gender norms and values was not only altering relations based on these but also establishing such changes as a new way of being and living within communities.

Interview with H

H: I am a child from parents who had problems because of war. I was born in 1971. My father died in 1972 because of his ethnicity. Mother told us we were orphans because dad had been killed for his ethnicity. We grew up in bad conditions, but I could study till the 10th grade. I was clever. But I was not happy of how I was directed. Because of ethnicity I was oriented to LP [Lycee Pedagogique—Primary school for Teachers]. I did not want to go there. I resisted and stayed at home. But mum insisted. I obeyed and went but I did not like that school. While I was in the second year of the school in 1993, the war broke out. I was in Kayanza. I am Hutu. They killed all Hutus who did not flee. I was saved. I was arrested; they wanted to burn me. I managed to escape. I left the school because many people died there, because I was Hutu I was not directed well and they wanted to kill me. I went back to school later but I was not proud of my studies. I finished in 1994. I found a job as a teacher in Muruta commune, near Kibira forest [primary base of the rebellion]. I used to walk to the school. I was living in parish lodging. My elder sister, a teacher at the same school, lived also there. Then the place was attacked and we fled. After we came back the place was attacked again. They killed 21 people that day. Those who escaped fled away; no one could find each other. Life was very bad because of poverty. Then I found my sister in 1997, we were the only ones survived from our group. We both found jobs as teachers. We were really suffering because of the recent past. Then we heard of a movement said to be trying to free Hutus. We were not happy with what was happening to us. I searched and I found the movement. I was not forced to join; I agreed with my sister on this, we wanted to help them [fighters]. So I went into the forest and went for military training. Military life was not easy. I had a tough life, very difficult life. The movement leader was Nyangoma at the time. Beside ethnic divide there was also regional divide. Because I was from the North, they beat me very badly. Then I was afraid and quit then came back to my elder sister. And we lived together for a while. She was not married yet. We both did not want to get married because the life was not good. Finally she was married in 1999 and I did in 2000. We were married almost in the same moment we were very close to each other. But it was accidental, it was not well planned. My husband did not know anything about my fighting past, and I knew nothing of his opinion. Progressively we became close and I opened up, I told him about the life with the movement as he was willing to support this ideal. In 2002, he agreed I could go back to the bush, although the war was near the end. My husband stayed at home. I stayed in the bush. Then quickly came peace agreement and they sent us to assembly points. After it was the demobilization and reintegration. I asked to be reintegrated in my old job. Then we were back in the community, we were perceived as violent, killers, and people were cold with us. I don't know how this will change.

INTERVIEWER: What is the situation now?

H: Things are changing very slowly day by day with regular contact. People continue to think demobilized combatants could not have good relations with their neighbors they see them as less than animals. I see we try hard we had hard life we are able to make great effort to have good relations with other people. People used to say that we are killers but you could see that we were not the first to do this we just tried to defend ourselves as we were constantly provoked for many years. Even before the killings occurred they kept saying that. When a murder happened they said it is the ex-combatants. Most of the time normal people commit those crimes. You know before ex-combatants came back in the community there were murders and theft.

Let me give you another example, on rape. People used to say that ex-combatants are responsible for all rapes. Even common criminals would hide themselves under this cover, as they know that people surely will blame ex-combatants for rapes and killings. People are likely to blame ex-combatants not acknowledging that usual criminals do that too. But really, many young girls had been raped, you could see this because they have babies while not being in marriage. This hurts us. Because having been in the military, we know what discipline is. Even one who had no personal discipline when s/he joined the military s/he had to change. War teaches you discipline you just can't behave as you want.

INTERVIEWER: Could you please elaborate the situation of ex-combatants? Why they are seen as criminals?

H: Yes. People just generalize and treat us as criminals. So as a woman they don't believe we were soldiers they say we were just "wives" for male soldiers. They say we are accustomed to uncontrolled sex life. This makes me sad. I am married. I can say that no one single man came to me in the bush for sexual relation. In military they have strong tough regulations. Even some, I would say, not proper men who could come into the military and keep having uncontrolled sexual life, they would have encountered many punishments to get them into the right behavior. Some individuals were having wild sexual life; they had to come back to discipline and follow regulation of the rebellion.

INTERVIEWER: How about this talk of rapes, could you say a bit more on this?

H: Of course it happened. It is normal. When men and women are together. … Even in normal life … yes it happened. When grown up men and women … they are natural needs—"besoins naturels." At the beginning it was not authorized to have couple life, but some did. After a period, leaders saw that it was natural they saw that they could not control it. They changed the rule. After that, when a man or a woman wanted to go into couple life with someone, they were asked to let it be known to the commandant. At that point they would become married. This was unofficially the marriage, but they were accepted as married. There were many cases of marriage like this. Many are still together.

INTERVIEWER: How did people get to know each other?

H: You could be in the same unit or be together working, fighting. There were no separation between men and women in the bush except for lodging. In lodging we had separated place for women.

INTERVIEWER: What about rape in the war?

H: When it happened either in the camp or during the fighting they just raped people. They never thought of HIV/AIDS. They just wanted to rape. For some men rape was just an objective … because it was a natural need. As a rule when a man took a woman this way, he had to keep her as "wife" [in the camp]. When they were both fighters they stayed together.

INTERVIEWER: How?

H: If threatened with a gun? No. There was no other way to stop it. If a man found opportunity, he found a woman and forced her into sex, she would not consider accusing him of rape. She would rather keep their relation secret. If she accused him of forcing her he would be sentenced to her as wife. There was no motivation for women to complain. This happened to unmarried women, never to a married woman. This was unthinkable [in the camps].

This was not really frequent. People were preoccupied with combat, they were busy they did not think of sex. They knew they could be attacked at any time. Commanders tried to really control people it was hard to find a moment to enter into matters of sex. May be because of this, when out in the battle field, they frequently raped women. They did not tell us about these officially. But they talked among themselves, secretly, they talked to their friends and at the end this was known to everybody. Men were proud of this.

Now we are out of rebellion. Both sides, rebels and the military [FAB], raped women. Soldiers are the same. May be FAB had leave time, while rebels did not. Rebels were in the bush with no regular contact with other people. In the bush, when they had opportunity they raped for sexual need. But military they had regular contact with other people and opportunity for normal sexual life. Military did rape for revenge. On the battle field rebels raped to satisfy their natural needs. They did not care about ethnicity of the women they raped. Then, military would come and if they were informed that rebels raped women from this ethnic group [Tutsi] they would consider to take revenge and rape rebel's people [Hutu].

INTERVIEWER: What was the situation in IDP camps?

H: FAB guarding IDP camps though that "Ahaa, our group is being killed … we are becoming fewer. We need to increase our numbers. They raped women in order to increase the number of their people, not necessarily for other reasons. Rebels raped women because they needed to satisfy natural needs, they did not think of ethnicity. Also battles usually happened during the night. It is hard to see ethnicity during the night; it is hard to see a woman is a Hutu or a Tutsi. FAB came and considered ethnicity. During the war families usually gathered in groups based on ethnicity in the hillsides. Then FAB came and raped Hutu girls to revenge. Soldiers treated people badly. Women were beaten, raped and killed. They did this also because of indiscipline.

INTERVIEWER: How do you think the gender relations changed?

H: In Burundian culture war is not for women it is not for women to take guns to live in the bush to kill people. Then the culture was broken apart, and women expanded quickly to do things they had to do. They were unprepared. Women had to change quickly and try to adapt. Before, men and women use to have distance among them. Then this usual distance between men and women was quickly suppressed. In the bush or in the camp we lived with men all around. We were together all the time. Because of this proximity between men and women, women became accustomed to this closeness, they started to talk, joke and play and this could easily lead to other things. War started this spread of HIV. The closeness is a factor for HIV. When you don't see a man, you may not think of them. But when you are together all the time, in direct contact, walking, sitting, the idea is there [sexual relations].

In looking at this interview, it is possible to identify a set of reference points for understanding the way gender and conflict interacted. H's gender position is underwriting her views. It is based on being a ranked female ex-combatant during the rebellion and attaining a particular position within the rebel ranks. In addition at the time of the interview, after the conflict, she was a senior civil servant in one of the ministries in Bujumbura. In her thinking, gender relations were considered not only according to inter-ethic division but also according to intra-ethnic gender relations and regional differences between ex-combatants. Furthermore, from her views on sexual violence it is possible to argue that intra-gender relations based on rank and age are important markers for understanding boundaries of gender relations that were dis-articulated and rearticulated in the conflict. The interview also highlights a set of processes influencing the instrumentalization of women that became major source of gender vulnerability during the conflict.

Her life story presents the overall impact that the context of conflict has on one woman's life. The conflicts from 1972 onwards set the socio-cultural and political context for her life and influenced the way she was treated. Once again the belonging via paternal lineage had an important impact. Another issue highlighted in the interview is the impact of conflict-related mobility on a person who was not within the traditional family unit. The initial move to join the rebellion might have been a survival act/mechanism. However, the reality once H joined was different. The critical issue here is the dif-ference between the way she talks about her experience during the rebellion before she completed her education and got married and afterwards, when she joined the rebellion a second time on more ideological grounds as a pro-fessional, after completing her education, and being married. There is a clear tension between her understanding of female ex-combatants' role in the con-flict and her engagement with the experiences of other women who were exposed to in her words the natural needs of men in the bush. At this point in the discussion her military and social positions seem to influence how she reflects on the past. There is a sense of an inevitability to the sexual violence in this context because of men's needs; she is implicitly also suggesting that under these conditions women had little to do. She refers to men's *natural needs*, which implies that these had to be addressed and women were power-less to do much. This inevitability was, as she points out, due to the proximity of being in the same place but also about the expected engagement between men and women. The reconfiguration of social relations in the conflict acted as a driver of change in gender relations. For women in the rebellion there was a dramatic change forcing them to alter their traditional position of being a woman framed by quietness and withdrawn attitudes. Here the observed change is in part a result of the erosion of the traditional spaces women occupied and the way their traditional positions were exploited used. Suddenly, they were in a particular public space created by the conflict where they were expected to assume roles they had not occupied before. The con-tours of H's interview provide insights about the conflict context and the vulnerabilities created for women, in particular for those women who were part of the rebellion. The latter indicates a disarticulation of traditional roles, which had implications for these women in the post-conflict context.

Interview with I

I: I am 31 and live in Ngozi commune. I am married and have one child. I was in the military—with the rebellion. I do my own business, the project started with the reinsertion allowance—to build a house on the family land here. I was born here. The money was used to finish the house. My project was to sell wheat flour, rice and different items from a shop but I sold it all to build the house. My wife used to sell small things [tomatoes] in the market. I have no job, but I recently passed the driver's test and I am waiting for the permit. So hoping to get a job as a taxi moto driver.

I was demobilized in 2005—June 23rd. Then with the first installment of the reinsertion money (300,000 BUF) I started to get material for the house like sheeting, bricks and began the building. I married in 2000 then two months after, I joined the rebellion.

INTERVIEWER: Could you tell us more about how you joined?)

I: My life was very bad. My family was very poor. Also there was fighting all around in the bush—neighbors suspected that I had collaborated with them. Police came and took me, I was beaten, I paid them and left. At the time if people suspected you they could kill you—I did not tell my wife or family, just went, they [rebels] accepted me. I integrated into the rebellion. And fought until the ceasefire, then demobilized and came home. At the time of demobilization, there was the option to join the military but I thought that my wife might long after me so I demobilized. After the ceasefire at the beginning people avoided me looking with a bad eye. They discriminated me before fighting so when I was back I thought I might take revenge. I did not take revenge. I tried to have good relations. Slowly, progressively it is alright.

When I was married I did not want to leave her in a rented house so I installed her with my parents. In time my brothers, sisters and cousins thought that she should go because after two years not coming back, they thought I might be dead. Not legally married. This was a factor for my relatives thinking to chase her away. They did not see me, may be because we were not legally married, they complained she should go. When I was back, I was in the same compound (we have a large compound) they gave me a plot near the street because I am the only son of my mother and they also gave land to my half-brother (my father's son from outside the home). I have five sisters, three are married, two are unmarried and at home-in school one in the 9th grade and the other one is 8th grade.

INTERVIEWER: What was it like in the bush?

I: I would not say it was good. It was very bad. We had tough military exercises and the food was very bad. We lived in forests, in swamps and had a very bad life. Sometimes I felt I should give up but thought that at home it was very unjust so I stayed. I stayed because of what I saw in the hillsides. It was not really for salary or medicine, it was for change. It was not the same for everyone. Some were told nice things about freeing the country. In the hillsides some thought of liberating the country for freedom. They were also told nice things about fighting, you would get money and other things. They had wrong ideas of the bush, there were many like this. Some feared battle and left. I see now that I am alive-thank God not because I am smart but because God saved me. Sometimes 10 went to fight and only three came back. The others were dead and we passed them running back-it was tough. We also saw some normal [non-armed civilians] people.

Some in the community collaborated with rebels. They would support us with food. It was difficult if you did not know each other. If a rebel goes into a community and someone would tell lies, saying that "wait here I will give you food" and then they went to the military to capture you. Sometimes in the hillsides, if you camp, you would find soldiers circled house to catch everyone. You then know that they told about us to the military. If the community caught rebels we were angry so we sometimes searched for them we caught the people from that community. We did not treat them badly—some became fighters or porters. This happened especially near the Kibara forest, some came freely.

INTERVIEWER: How about women?

I: We had female fighters. I saw many female combatants joining us. You would see in the night, young women coming with food on their heads and they did not return. We thought they came from nearby communities. Some came willingly, but not really willingly. They were forced. They arrived, we trained them and some became fighters.

INTERVIEWER: How were they forced?

I: You know, in the community [rebel], there was someone responsible to collect food. If there were not enough rebels to bring food they forced people [locals] to help. Some became fighters, some did not. They go back and become responsible for food collection in the community. They had to be either fighters or food collectors. In the camps there were two parts. We lived in bunkers for men and across from women. If you were caught going across to the women's part, you could lose your rank from 1st to 2nd class for example. It was not possible for unranked (2nd rank) to go to women. So for ranked men it was possible to court women and some got pregnant and gave birth and sometimes women were ranked. It was unthinkable for unranked men, it was tough. If caught he was beaten to half-dead so others did not think of going. It was secret even ranked men hid, they did not want to lose rank. A woman would think twice before complaining because she knew that she would be punished for the initial relationship. Sometimes when fighting rebels, or when it was time to go to the battlefield, some stole, some broke into homes and raped women. You know we had camps and positions in the bush. Some fighters leave the camp and force women.

INTERVIEWER: Was there any discussion of HIV/AIDS?

I: [Shakes his head] Fighters were not in the mood to think about that. They said "we are dead" there is no death more present than a gunshot—they did not think of it as important. No one talked about it. I knew it existed but during the war no one talked about until the demobilization camps.

INTERVIEWER: Was there a talk about condoms?

I: No, never. Sometimes there was suspicion of HIV in one or another.

INTERVIEWER: How?

I: You know male fighters did not trust female fighters. Because they suspected some women were not shy or proper they went easily with men. We saw chatting and laughing. We saw women went with many so we thought. ... Among men they would sit and chat—they say may be she is dangerous, may be HIV+ but they did not really talk about HIV/AIDS. Then they would avoid her. She still has sex with other fighters but in secret.

INTERVIEWER: Were there married women?

I: Yes, they were known to be married even if unofficially. They were respected as such. These kinds of women were respected as wives. Single women were not respected, so could be talked about. Men sometimes fought over women. But not between men and women they would have been punished. These were generally insults and not really fights. Fights were sometimes because of theft. If one came in to the bunker and saw that something was missing, they fought. I never saw men fighting over in the battlefield.

In this interview "I" provides a view from the position of a young rebel within the troops rather than a ranking officer. On the one hand his interview confirms some of the issues raised by H in relation to women's conditions in the rebellion. On the other hand he qualifies some of the interpretations on the state of women provided by H based on her position. "I" gives nuanced understanding of structural gender relations in the conflict. Furthermore, his reflections on his own life and how he joined the rebellion reveal the circumstances under which women who were left behind had to live. The conditions present when he joined and his life under arms draw attention to the pressure young men were exposed to by their communities. In his case he indicates that it was safer for him to join the rebellion rather than live outside it and to come under suspicion from the community. The interview also sheds light on the circumstances of women who were left behind by their husbands or fathers without much paternal protection. Here the circumstances of women were made worse by a changing social context trying to legitimate intra-family practices according to the existing gender relations where the protection and support of the husband creates the link between their wives and their families. These issues are highlighted in various ways. Initially one of the central issues here is the way traditional marriage is under pressure and pushed to its limits when men were not around to legitimate it. I's concern about his wife while he was away was clearly justified as his family tried to distance themselves from the wife. This was partially driven by intra-family resource allocation priorities as there was another brother in the family from the father's extra-marital relationship. The fact that this problem was discussed by many of our interviewees points out how the conflict exposed the limits of traditional marriage very sharply.

Later in his discussion of women in the rebellion, "I" provides a picture from a different angle, i.e., from the angle of women who found themselves in the middle of the rebellion. Some of these women were engaging with rebels to provide resources for them, while others were joining to fight. In both cases the initial processes of becoming part of the rebel group was dangerous and women suffered. I's discussion confirms H's point about the separation between male and female combatants and the potential for severe punishments. However, his view also suggests that at the lower ranks men were able to use the potential of punishment as leverage to have sexual relations. He does not say much about the circumstances of sexual violence outside the camps.

In relation to women who join the rebellion, there is also the question of motivation. There is a degree of voluntarism in both I's interview and in H's commentary about her own past. However, this idea of voluntarism needs to be unpacked. Two interviewees (W and X) have provided insights on this. Both were female ex-combatants with the rebellion and came back from the bush with young children. Both were in a group discussion and wanted to talk to us outside group at the end:

> In 1996 I was at the school, 7th grade. They [rebel fighters] used to come and take students; some students were killed and some were forced to follow them. They used to write a letter to the school and tell the students that they will come. Then they come and fetch you. If you think this, you would go voluntarily. If you go under force, those would be treated badly. I joined by myself. Others were already kidnapped. In the letter they would write and say which way you need to follow and say you come this far and we will wait for you (around Kibera). When you arrive there were military exercises, we were not happy but it was forced. It was not a happy time we were raped and forced [to have sex]. We fought we had many problems. At the time of demobilization we were offered the option to join the new military. But it had been long time in the bush we did not accept.
>
> I was in the 6th grade in Mutumba commune. When the war broke out, they came and took the girls. They were writing letters to the head-master or to the students directly. When we arrived in the school we would receive the letters. Many hand written letters spread around the school. They would kidnap one student, she will give those names and they [fighters] will come with a list and drop the list. When they come back there would be a copy of the list. They came to take students on the list, during the day they say come and meet us in the bush. We lived in the bush, life was very difficult. They raped us, we didn't know then, we did not know who they were. They told us that it was a military command that we had to have sex. Rebel soldier would order you to go with him. There were different men ranked or not. We had this problem at the beginning we did not know who is ranked and who is not to order you. In time we realized who is ranked and who is not. Then you could say no

and refuse to have sex but then you had to accept to beaten. It meant that that you did not respect orders and you had to be punished. The relationship depended on his (combatant) own mood, he could have kept you for a long time, up to 2 years. We also saw some change as the time went on some men kept long term partners.

These two interviews provide insights to an important process whereby the rebellion was able to convince young women to join them. Here the question of voluntarism is contentious. The interviews reveal clearly that the women's decisions to join were taken under duress with an evident threat clear from what was happening around them in their schools. It is also clear that armed men manipulated women's existing subservient behavior towards men in public. This was also the case after women were brought to camps where their subservience together with the threat of violence was used for sexual abuse. These reflections also provide some context to H's view on the sexual relations she discusses in her interview. Men were able to instrumentalize traditional attitudes to subvert the existing regulations for punishment. While low-ranking fighters resorted to these methods to take advantage of women, higher ranks were practically free to do as they wished.

The implication of this for gender relations is dramatic. Intra-ethnic sexual violence was severe and persistent. It was dependent on the way existing gender relations were manipulated to benefit men in what they considered to be opportunistic situations. It also seems that the long time spent isolated in the bush amplified men's behavior. At the same time, in line with I's reflections, these interviews show that the modality of traditional marriage was being used to justify sexual relations in the rebellion without providing any ability for women to enforce these arrangements either during or after the conflict.

Another important aspect of these interviews is the way they unpack the relationship between low- and high-ranking rebels in the conflict. It seems that women's bodies were utilized to maintain the hierarchy and reinforce power relations between different ranks. The modus operandi of this process was to use the women's gender position to objectify them as a kind while regulating access to their bodies according to the military hierarchy developed during the rebellion. Paradoxically, women were being pushed to do things they had never done before, yet the measure of what they were doing remained referenced to their traditional gender positions. In other words, their experiences were not a real concern for the men. They were living through the rebellion. At the same time many of the women's experiences were going to mark them as unacceptable in their own communities after the conflict. Their past would be evaluated according to the ongoing gender considerations.

Interview with J

J: I was born in Mwumba Commune. My mother and father are from different ethnic groups. You know war was about ethnicity. Father is Hutu and mother is Tutsi. In 1993 Tutsi were targeted to be killed. Mother was targeted to be killed. So we fled to Rwanda. Even in Rwanda some Burundians were really after us to find and kill her. Us young boys we tried to protect her. They even came to our house where we were staying. Hutu refugees in Rwanda were after mother to kill her. Then we came back to Burundi in 1994 to our land in Mwumba. But everything was destroyed. Then the political situation began to be very bad for us in Mwumba. People were not only after mother, but they were also after father saying "You are Hutu, you married a Tutsi, you are not a good Hutu, and your kids are not really Hutu." We were attacked twice. Then we moved to the town. So my elder brother and younger sister and I were able to go back to the school. Because of poverty I had to help the family. I just stopped my studies in the 8th grade. Then I joined the army. After the three months training, I went to fight. Both parents were jobless and the family lived in very bad condition. Elder brother and young sister were kept in the school. I supported the family. Some finished their studies. One is at the university here. Another one joined the army after the secondary school. I am still single now because I need to support the family. I spent eight years in the army and quitted. Before that I was badly wounded on the right leg. I was in bed for six months and then it healed and I went to my job. Then in July 2005 I thought of quitting as they asked for volunteers to be demobilized. I wanted to quit as I joined the army because of poverty and lack of security. At the time the situation was improving and I decided to quit. I talked to my parents. They agreed and tried to find another way of getting resources. Also before quitting I paid off a bank credit 200,000 BIF which I used to buy a plot of land in Ngozi town. In February 2006 I was demobilized. Then with my reinsertion package I began building my own house. It is finished now.

There is usual stigmatization of ex-combatants. When there is a theft somewhere, people blame ex-combatants. When the inquiry is done, the find no ex-combatants is involved. Suspicion remains. For female ex-combatants the situation is not the same. Most of them here in the town are married to important or rich men. In this commune there are five female ex-combatants: two were students and married to high ranking soldiers. There is another one who has a telephone shop in the market. There was another one who was known to be HIV-infected and died. This woman with the telephone shop had problems because she had many relations the bush. She was with high ranking FDD officer—Colonel. She is here, he left her while she was pregnant. She is now married to someone else.

INTERVIEWER: Did you talk about HIV/AIDS in the military?

J: No, there was no time, we just talked about the war. We only had information afterwards in the demobilization camps but it was not enough. Rebels did not have any information either. You know, during the war, everything was about the war only. For me, let's say of 100 days of military life I did not get even 5 days for rest. I only got a rest when I was shot and went to the hospital. It was not possible to talk or even to think about HIV/ AIDS. Even in the hospital I never talked about it with anyone. All the time we talked about the war and different things about it.

INTERVIEWER: Did soldiers have girlfriends?

J: Yes, but not really girlfriends, not from military camps. When we were sent to military positions in the field, soldiers took [had sex with] young girls who lived nearby. Soldiers were usually sent to places where people were grouped in camps. When they were fighting in the bush they could have a day out. Then three or four men could go together looking for girls. Then they would take young girls. They could take different girls, or all of them take [have sex] the same girl going in one after another. This happened for many soldiers many times. As I saw among my friends, it happened regularly. For example one of those deceased I told you about, was born in Mivo. We were together and we joined the army at the same time. We were in Bujumbura Rural, near Sororezo, then in Nyabiraba, then in Kabarore commune in Kayanza. Of course it is hard to know where he was infected and from which women. But I would say he was infected in Kabarore. Another one, who was not demobilized, is now dead. He was infected in the same place in Kabarore. Then we were moved to Bujumbura Rural, I don't remember exactly where may be in Isale commune, then Gasenyi and then Mutimbuzi. Each three months we were moved to another military position. And other soldiers came to replace us, while we moved to another place to replace a unit that gets out, and so on. Some individuals from our group or from previous group in that place were infected some of the women they visited were infected. Infected people went all over the place, moved and left behind infected women, and infected other women in other places. Those women had new soldiers coming to them and more people were infected, see …

I was in the 4th commando battalion with green berets we had a strong reputation of being the best fighters. So we were sent into the hardest places and we were moved often. For example in Nyabunyegeri, near Kibira forest, we were sent many times for fighting to this place. Another example, we were sent to hold another position near Teza (Bukeye Commune) near the forest. We used to fight the rebels in the forest. A unit kept the place for a moment, two months, fighting heavily, and was then sent back to a more calm and normal military position. Back in that situation, it was possible to see civilians, we had money and soldiers easily go to women. We had money, not much money, but some. We used to court women and pay them. Men would go knowingly to the same woman all of them three, four, this increased the risk of HIV.

Rebels were in the bush, they had women with them. They could have sexual relations. Also during the fighting they went to places and raped women, a group of rebels could rape the same woman. There were ambushes against cars and buses on the roads. They then killed men and raped women. All these could increase the risk of HIV infection. With rebels sexual relations were likely to be forced, after fighting, we saw many women raped by rebels, many women were complaining about being raped. With FAB we had some money and in military positions we had possibilities, to go have a beer, to give a bottle or two to woman we would than negotiate sex.

INTERVIEWER: Did people use condoms?

J: No, not many soldiers were informed about condoms. There were no condoms in battlefield. Using condom this could not happen easily … you know our life during the fighting … I can't tell you how tough it was, we carried just few things with us you could not keep things like even a condom in your pockets, you could not think of a condom at a time like that. People just had sex.

Women could not discuss these things … in a situation when many men were running after women. You know in IDP camps, displaced women were like in prison, they could not go to the fields to get food, they sometimes go cultivate their land and come back to the IDP camp for the night. Their lives did not allow them to ask for condom. They were very poor and weak. There was no room for negotiation, as they feared men to treat them badly.

For soldiers there was both sex for money and forced sex. Also offering beer helped soldiers' "success" in sexual relations. You know sexual relations came in different ways. One young soldier, married, had not yet had time to go back home, saw a friend going on leave. He give this friend some money and say "Please give this money to my wife when you arrive." The soldier friend then would find the wife. She would ask "how is my husband?" He would say "He is well. He gave message for you let's go for a beer and I will tell you." He would then go out for a beer with this young woman and they get drank and would have sex. Another HIV risk.

Soldiers were more powerful than the Bashingantahe, than the hillside chief or the IDP camp chief. Women treated soldiers nicely as they had guns and they were protecting the camps. Some women might have thought that these soldiers were our protectors. What can I do if not accept what he asks? He protects me know if I don't accept him he may not protect me. Women feared when they accepted to have sex. They had accepted sexual relations they would not have done in other situations. Sometimes our military positions were near to IDP camps. Sometimes there was conflict in a camp and they came to us to settle the problem. Soldiers seemed to have enough authority to settle conflict more quickly. They preferred soldiers to the civilian authority. We were interested in this as we got money and beer.

The interview with J points out once again a life course influenced by the conflict in the country. In this case he observes the complex mobility patterns created by the conflict. His parent's story shows a pattern of escape out of the country and then back into it, a pattern which was experienced by many others. Furthermore, it shows a pattern of conflict creeping into private lives. His reflections on military life unpacks the mobility associated with military deployment and their aims. At the same time the story is about people's movements within the country due to conflict. His story gives insights about one of the central mechanisms creating pressure on gender relations: the movement of people across the country. It had emerged at the juncture of people's internal displacement and the regular movement of rebels and the military. This mechanism illustrates the context within which socialization between soldiers and other people took place and how vulnerabilities to HIV risks were created. Here the pattern is different from the rebels. J is talking about the government's regular army in which sexual relations took place with women from outside the military structure. He talks about different kinds of relations. Some were with sex-workers who were paid for sex. It is clear that this group of women were particularly vulnerable as they were specifically targeted by groups of soldiers. Others were with women who were engaging in transactional sex. This behavior might have also been opportunistic from the women's perspective, since the availability of resources to the soldiers made them an attractive resource base. Here the issue of provision of beer is important, since selling the beer they received from a sexual encounter was a potential income stream for them. The move from transactional opportunistic sexual encounters to sex-work could also be seen as a process in which women were gradually socialized as the conflict continued. In J's comments it is possible to observe implicitly that he is talking about how available women were to soldiers' advances. This availability and the new way of socializing need to be understood in relation to the social change women experienced due to the conflict. They were left behind and sometimes forced to leave their homes. The existing conflict conditions that created pressure on gender relations forcing women to move also pressurized them into sexual encounters with important follow-on implications for them. The commentary about IDP camps is also informative in showing the kinds of gender vulnerabilities that were experienced by women who were trying to remain in some kind of community context. However, the nature of the IDP camps meant that women and soldiers were positioned in constant close proximity in a dramatically unbalanced power context. The particular context of IDP camps exacerbated the general gender vulnerability of women as a survival calculus combined with powerlessness came into play when they engaged with soldiers. The changing nature of military deployment is also an important factor here. The prolonged conflict meant that soldiers moved more and more across the country. These movements created a social context driven by the soldiers' needs which interacted with women's survival needs, when considered together this led to a vulnerability to HIV risks.

During a discussion in Bujumbura Rural at a meeting of local group of HIV+ people from different communes, participants linked some of the concerns on conflict highlighted above with HIV. It was clear that even for those who did not participate in the conflict, as combatants or in other ways, displacement affected everyone. The group included five people and one of them was male, K a widower, in his mid-30s at the time with five children. The others were women who were also widows with between two to five children.

They are all involved in a local HIV information group and talked about the HIV/AIDS issues in their own communities.

K: During the war people were fleeing, they were in despair, especially women. Women slept with men for money which they needed to live. This propagated HIV. This is how HIV spread during the war. I had a second wife, she was looking for money, because of war she took me. I fled to Tanzania, then to Congo (DRC) and back through Nyanza Lac—I knew I was HIV +. She went with other men, that is how I became infected. My first wife then separated from me.

L: People fled due to war. Even married people became sick and may be they gave birth to a child who was stillborn. People then tested here, then in Bujumbura, then here again. There was no treatment. I have no house, or land, life is hard.

M: People say my husband was HIV+, I lived in Gatumba [a camp on the border with DRC] and he raised cattle. When I became ill, I came here and tested. He became infected because he bought cows in Kanyosha [in Bujumbura].

N: Many people are infected. It is not just because of war, but the war made it worse. Poverty was also a major factor, your children are hungry and you do what you need to do to get food for them. HIV is spreading, we are vulnerable. Many people are having sex, many times, husbands are problem. I fled to Nyanza Lac, my husband died there, then I came home (back here) because of hunger and poverty. HIV was not just caused by the war, people are tempted by sex, men are not real men, they are not responsible, they infected many women and children. Here in Kabezi, many many are infected.

O: I agree with N. HIV is another war. Women were not responsible and now they are infected. I was never out of the house yet I am infected. Now this is another war. War and HIV – both are wars but I don't know how they both came about. I did not think of condoms because I am a good woman. I stay at home, so in my mind, there was no need to think of condoms. HIV was also passed because some women were raped. Being grouped in camps also increased HIV.

N: Some were infected while fleeing the war.

M: My husband fled two times, the first time he came home he was single. The second time he brought home another wife. Many became infected this way because men had sex with others.

These reflections show how the peoples' movements created vulnerabilities both for themselves and for others. Here, a notable issue is the difference between men's and women's movements. In most cases it seems husbands' movements were significant in terms of creating vulnerability for their wives. The case of K, in particular, is interesting as independent of his mobility he seems to blame his second wife for his infection. He does not provide an account of his other sexual liaisons in his movements. L's comment is implicitly engaging with the men's behavior outside the family and how this might have impacted their wives. M and O are indicating that they were infected because of their husbands who were traveling and having sexual relations. They were also palpably surprised when they realized they were infected. This discussion provides a picture of displacement within the general population. The mobility of men meant that women were gradually made vulnerable both within and outside family structures, even if husbands were not part of the conflict as fighters or soldiers.

Conclusion

The aim of this chapter was to understand the way various dynamics were set into motion by the conflict and created the particularities of this conflict that interacted with the existing gender norms in Burundi. In many of the interviews, interviewees reflecting on their experiences consider conflict to be correlated with HIV. The conflict provides a cognitive lens for them to explain and understand how they either became HIV+ themselves or how it has become prevalent in their communities. However, most seem to be implicitly talking about the gender relations they live with as setting the conditions for HIV risks.

The impacts of the conflict on gender relations were experienced in differentiated spaces. Many families were broken. Men were joining the conflict which put traditional marriages into question. Intra-household resource conflicts exposed the limits of traditional marriage to protect the women who were left behind. The stress put on traditional marriage meant that many women were made homeless and many young women were left without paternal protection. Yet they all had to survive. They engaged with other men in public to support themselves. This no doubt changed women's behavior. Furthermore, as the conflict developed into a prolonged process, women without paternal protection or fixed home became vulnerable to being incorporated into the conflict. The context of the camps as pointed out above by a number of the interviewees created another impact. The space created by proximity, the anxiety of fighting, and the potential for imminent sexual abuse put gender relations under pressure, particularly at the expense of women. In addition, the overarching gender governance that valorized particular traits of assertive masculinity meant that men also had to act and perform in ways they would not have done before the conflict. As a result, while women's traditional gender roles were capitalized to assert the masculine order, they were forced to assume and perform different roles within the rebellion. The sexual abuse and the positions that were defined as bush wives evolved into systematic behavior. In some ways this also indicates an altering position of masculinity. Gradually men who had families before the conflict had to find justifications that underwrote their continuing relationships with particular women. At the same time women, outside the camps, who happened to be in the vicinity of armed groups, were also open to abuse. Conversely, the women who sought protection in IDP camps were also vulnerable. Many women found themselves in abusive contexts. Nonetheless, it appears that many changed their behavior to survive and engaged in transactional sex. The complexity of these changes represent inter- and intra-ethnic patterns of violence which are also informed by age, regional, educational, and wealth differences. Gender analysis also allows these to be considered in a more focused manner than the way international policy discussion frames these complexities under a bland category of "ethnic violence," which arguably reduces the nature of violent behavior to just one of the possible relationships. The discussion presented above fits well with Daley's (2008: 110) assessment that "a vast proportion of violence takes place between the same ethnic group." The sexual violence which is discussed by many of the interviewees suggests an inherent link between the way behavior is governed by gender norms and how these were manipulated during the conflict.

The discussions in this chapter could easily be interpreted as a way of looking at a familiar story in relation to conflict, women, and violence (Bennett *et al.* 1995; Mertus 2000; Jacobs *et al.* 2000; Moser and Clark 2001; Lindsey 2001; Rehn and Sirleaf 2002). However, the material presented in this chapter, and that included in the earlier chapters, presents a much more nuanced and complicated situation. These narratives unpack the way *being a woman* and *being a man* were framed according to particular gender governance. They also indicate how the conflict altered this particular governance. It is also clear that the gender governance informing relations during the conflict was informed by relations that were related to intra-gender differences depending on the regional, ethnic, and educational differences among women and also among men. The change during the conflict was also due to the way women were actively engaging with their conditions to maintain their lives. It is clear from the discussions above that women developed many survival strategies which created a new way of being a woman. For instance the reflections on the way women sometimes transitioned from being food carriers to fighters indicate a significantly different way of engaging with their gender roles which traditionally prescribed subservience. These kinds of survival strategies undoubtedly presented a major challenge to the assertive masculinity of many rebels. While women changed their behavior to deal with the circumstances, the measure for judging their behavior remained referenced to the traditional gender governance. This was also the masculine reaction to these changes influencing their self-perception underwritten by the traditional roles assigned to them in gender governance. This allowed, in the eyes of many men, further abuse and violence to be acceptable for those women whom they considered unworthy. The same process and the resulting experience of women had complicated women's lives after the conflict when they were trying to normalize their conditions. These observations agree with Handrahan's observation that in post-conflict context "the national patriarchy reasserts itself" (2004: 436). However, here this issue needs to be considered with more critical understanding of how far patriarchal norms and values were part of women's lives during the conflict. The absence of a male figure from the context of family or community in the case of Burundi did not necessarily mean freedom. There is no doubt that many had to survive on their own and find adoptive ways to engage with the conflict context. However, many of these experiences that were shared do not indicate a picture of empowerment, particularly in relation to the overarching patriarchal context. Another indicator of this is linked with how women's experiences during conflict resulted in creating very limited benefits to them, in most cases depending on their education and their links to their male relations. I will turn to this in the next chapter.

4 HIV/AIDS in people's lives

This chapter focuses on how and what people, both combatants and non-combatants, thought about HIV and AIDS during the conflict and in the transition period at the end of the conflict. The aim of the chapter is to understand and consider the mechanisms relating to conflict and HIV in people's lives. This is a central missing piece in most of the discussions that consider the relationship between conflict and HIV. The discussion so far has considered gender relations as one of the central mechanisms through which the interaction between conflict and HIV is regulated. The previous chapters have discussed the way gender governance creates vulnerabilities to HIV risks during conflict.

The relationship between conflict and HIV is not simply assumed due to the disruptions created by conflict and observing incidents of HIV during the conflict. The occurrence of any conflict does not necessarily mean that people will get HIV. The argument is about the structural importance of gender governance and how it provides mechanisms for particular vulnerabilities to emerge for HIV risks. Therefore, the issue is not about the inevitability of HIV spread in the conflict context but rather about how vulnerability becomes a possibility depending on the gender relations in a given context. Here another issue is about HIV awareness and its influence on the way people acted: how far HIV was a part of, for instance, the cognitive world of combatants. While the gendered mechanisms make people exposed to HIV risks, it is also important to understand how people who were in the conflict considered these risks. It is not about whether HIV as a disease existed during the conflict and impacted people's lives. The issue is whether HIV as an idea and part of the knowledge repertoire existed to influence people's behavior. This is important for understanding how HIV spreads both in conflict and after the conflict. This chapter, first, looks at HIV awareness that existed among the combatants during the conflict and, second, it focuses on the Decommissioning, Demobilization and Reintegration (DDR) process, with specific attention to the circumstances of combatants in demobilization camps where they were given HIV/AIDS training. These camps acted as places of transformation for people to become civilian before they were discharged for reintegration at the end of the conflict. Therefore, they represent important places where the actual change on ID cards from combatants to civilians had to accompany cognitive change to engage with life after the conflict.

Gradual fading of HIV from the minds

The interviews reported in the last chapter touched on some of these issues. In particular, they reported experiences which in their minds created vulner-abilities to HIV among many men and women across the country. For instance, J talked about how conflict made it impossible to think about HIV while observing many possible avenues for HIV transmission. This was also in line with the reflection of "I," who pointed that sometimes combatants thought someone might be HIV+, but they did not really talk about it. The interaction between conflict processes and what little people knew about HIV meant that in the conflict period that knowledge gradually disappeared from people's minds. The reflections in the HIV+ group were also about the possi-ble pathways for HIV risk. In most of these reflections it was the intersection of various conflict-related social processes and gender governance that was considered to create vulnerability to HIV risks. As mentioned by one of the interviewees in the first chapter, many HIV/AIDS interventions stopped in Burundi with the 1993 conflict. What were the implications of this for people in thinking and acting during the conflict?

We had a discussion with two ex-combatants P (who was 24 at the time of the interview) and R (who was 40 at the time of the interview) in Makamba. Their reflections presented a timeline with which one could locate the HIV discussion. We could consider the changing nature of social relations and the places within which these changes took place. Importantly these places included demobilization camps at the end of the conflict.

P: In 1993, 95, 96 there was no HIV here, no information. When I returned in 2005 HIV/AIDS was visible. During the war, people were grouped in camps guarded by soldiers, soldiers had sex with girls, they did not care, they just had sex. Refugees and population movement increased HIV.

R: The war increased the spread of HIV. In cities, before fleeing, there was not much HIV. But by 2002 and 2003 many people were infected. There were many raped both in the bush and camps. Those infected became upset and under the pretext of war they raped people. Many men left for Tanza-nia and their wives stayed here, but sometimes they might have seen each other. Poverty was huge, so people moved to Tanzania. In Tanzania some women had sex for money some were raped when they went far from the camp looking for firewood.

P: In the bush having sexual relations was highly punished, it was better to kill than to rape. Some combatants had wives in the camp but they were eventually sent away because they were distracting. If you were infected it would be hard to fight until the end of the war. In demobilization camp we saw images and information about HIV, some went voluntarily for testing.

R: We had HIV training in Demobilization Camp but not enough it was useful but we still need more training. If you don't regularly hear about it you lose it. HIV/AIDS discussion has decreased, now people stop talking about it.

The discussion here indicates how HIV awareness over time disappeared from the conflict context. This created a perspective within the conflict in which HIV was ignored or assumed to be non-existent. The next time anyone openly had any discussion of the disease was in the demobilization camps.

In the following discussion the extent of this disappearance is unpacked. This is reported at a discussion with four female ex-combatants in Mugara, the part when they were asked if they knew about HIV during the war. All four answered at the same time saying *No* and added that there *was no information on HIV during the war*. One of them elaborated the statement:

> There was total disorder, people who were grouped increased HIV/AIDS. Women were raped when looking for firewood near the camps or in the fields or at their home. When women were raped there was no justice. In camps there was no food, no water, no information on HIV and people had sex all the time.

No doubt the unavailability of information was an important problem in the context of changing social relations that were creating more and more dispersed and multi-partnered sexual relations. The question, however, that needs to be asked is also about whether pre-1993 sensitization in Burundi had any impact on those who were exposed to it. If we go back to the interview with H, a ranking ex-combatant, she argued that:

> There was no occasion to talk about HIV in the camp. The main preoccupation was fighting. There was only time for military questions. There was no time to think about and follow HIV/AIDS-related information. This was the same in demobilization camps we only had a day on HIV/AIDS, not much to think about these issues. We were preoccupied about our next steps and what we will do once we are out of demobilization camps.

There was a similar reflection in J's interview where he talked about HIV as something he noticed in his fellow combatants and in the way they might have been infected. Once asked whether HIV was discussed, his response was:

> No there was no time, we just talked about the war. We only had information after the war, in the demobilization camp, but it was not enough. Rebels did not have any information. You know during the war everything was about the war only.

I's reflections also provided insight on this aspect of his life during the conflict. When asked whether they talked about HIV/AIDS during the war he said that:

> Fighters were not in the mood to think of that. They said that 'we are dead', there is no death more present than a gunshot ... they did not think of its importance. No one talked about it. I knew it existed but during the conflict never talked about it.

Another angle to this debate was highlighted in a discussion with a married ex-combatant couple who were in the rebellion together. In the discussion the husband pointed out that during the war:

> When men left the head of household role was broken, because of lack of trust. Some men closed their eyes, it was hard to get tested, broken homes increased the risks of HIV. Fighters 'looked' to see if a girl was 'healthy' if they looked healthy they had sex ... only after they saw HIV.

His wife added that:

> The war pushed the poverty [higher], people also missed HIV sensitization ... during the conflict you could really only hear about it on the radio and not everyone had radios.

The view emerging from these accounts together with others is that during the conflict HIV/AIDS was not targeted or brought to the attention of the combatants. Whatever information they might have had at the beginning of the conflict gradually disappeared or remained as a marginal or a non-issue in their everyday lives. Here age is also an important factor. Those who joined the rebellion at a young age would have missed sensitization material from before 1993 and thus would have had no knowledge of the disease. This also raises a question about the responsibility and the role of higher ranks to inform their rebel groups on HIV. The attitudes towards the possibility of HIV risk was also part of the conflict mind-set which focused on immediate mortal danger. One important implication of this is how the imminence of fighting influenced combatants' approach to sex. They wanted to take all possible opportunities that presented sexual encounter before potentially becoming a war casualty. In these calculations HIV did not seem to be a reference point. The gendered implications of this were calamitous.

Was the situation different in the regular army? It was one thing not to have any discussion of HIV in the rebellion as they lived mostly in the bush and camps. One might have expected more direct engagement with HIV in the army. Unfortunately, the story there was also not very positive. In an interview with S, a high-ranking member of the military personnel who left the military for other services in 2004, she talked about the absence of any concern for HIV during the conflict:

S: I see many women in the police coming from rebel groups, I see them they are always pregnant but they don't seem to think about HIV. I tried to talk to them but did not get support to develop the project.

INTERVIEWER: How was the situation with the army?

S: Before I was in the military training college there was sensitization. The officers were trained for sexual behavior in particular (but not really focusing on HIV). If you compare the time I entered (in 1993) and the present, many officers are infected now (many go out of the country to be tested). During the conflict this kind of sensitization did not continue. I don't think so, soldiers were in different places, difficult to reach places. If you see the way soldiers are getting married [she means the traditional marriage here] one understands that they are not sensitized. For instance, you see young soldiers in IDP camps or stationed camps near them [IDP camps] they take wives and some of these women follow them after they moved to a different place. There was promiscuity with the soldiers. I was in Bujumbura with many friends. Here we talked about HIV we listen to radio so we were educated people we could get informed. But as soldiers we were not really sensitized because of the conflict. After the ceasefire I am not sure they sensitized people. There is no sensitization in the police up to today. It is a subject that is abandoned today.

INTERVIEWER: Could you please say a bit more about the IDP issue you mentioned?

S: Sexual relations were frequent in IDP camps, I had many people coming to me complaining about soldiers' behavior. Displaced people were very poor. And soldiers benefitted from this. They raped people. What I saw in the conflict was that soldiers changed their behavior. You would see them doing things and don't understand why. I saw some of these through the complaints we had. You could also hear women on the radio complaining.

It is clear that the army's engagement with HIV was also patchy. Rank and location did matter and made differences to what people knew. The difficulty presented in this interview is the lack of organizational engagement with HIV. The fact that S was educated in Bujumbura meant that she had a community outside the army to engage in informative discussions. The same social context was not available to many soldiers who were young, from rural areas, and also spent most of their military experiences outside of Bujumbura and of the other urban areas. By being in the army their social context was confined within their groups and the people they met in the areas where they were deployed. Here, the possibility of an alternate social space where one could have considered discussing HIV and reflected on its implications was unrealistic. An interesting aspect of S's remarks is the way she confirms that radio was an important part of communication. As mentioned before, people talked about HIV on the radio in addition to voicing their complaints about different groups. Questions about the reach of these programs in the bush and camps as well as the availability of radios remain crucial. At the end of the conflict, both army and the rebels still had little engagement with HIV.

These reflections on the conflict context underline how risky it was to be in the conflict from the HIV point of view. This is, of course, compounded by the gender vulnerabilities resulting in differentiated outcomes for different gender groups who were part of the conflict. Undoubtedly the end of the conflict and the possibility of leaving this context behind was very important for people. This was also very important for development of HIV interventions for dealing with the risks highlighted up to now. For example, a social integration specialist felt that coming out of the conflict was central in terms of HIV risks:

> They [combatants] never talked about HIV/AIDS during the war. Some ex-combatants had some little information before demobilization. During the war HIV/AIDS was not an important subject to talk. During their stay in the demobilization camps they had information on HIV/AIDS and they reflected on how they were engaged in high risk lives during the conflict.

The situation during the conflict for soldiers and rebels was also the function of the dislocation from family and community relations in camps and in the bush. The prolongation of this dislocation generated a different kind of dynamic for social relations. The dislocation created over time a differentiated perception of time and space to people's lives. Their time horizons were changed in terms of their own lives. The social context was powered and maintained by the ever-present urgency of fighting. This urgency was intimately associated with the likelihood of death. In addition to the time factor the space was cognitively framed by the imminence of fighting. Physical space also created a particular kind of sociability. Here the issue was how many soldiers and rebels had to construct personal lives that were constantly in public. This was divergent from the context of lives habitually spent in communities and households. Even with the gender constraints discussed in the earlier chapters, the traditional context of a household in a community would have afforded more privacy for many people. Thus, these new dynamics of time and space shaped people's subjectivities. In other words, subjectivities were shaped by displacement and movement. In their behavior these subjectivities reasserted the time and space frameworks which were instrumental in their creation in the first place.

The intersection between this time and space framework and gender governance created a dynamic assertion of a kind of hyper-patriarchy, which in turn created a cycle of reproduction of the types of behavior reported by the interviews. In this cycle of reproduction, gender norms underwrote the traditional gender governance, for example, the expected subservence of women became sharply interpreted and deployed to exploit women. At the same time, the public nature of performance of this kind of behavior meant that men had to perform patriarchal norms and observe their boundaries to be accepted in this constraint context. This situation closed down any possible negotiation of gender norms more generally. It is at this juncture that HIV becomes a structurally contentious issue. While it is common sense to under-stand that the nature of the conflict made any new HIV interventions difficult, the reasons behind not informing combatants, rebels in particular, within the existing knowledge available by 1993 becomes an issue. Arguably, one expla-nation for the latter case is the development of this particular conflict-related subjectivity with its hyper-patriarchal gender framing. Engaging with HIV information and sensitization would have required the authorities to unpack not only the traditional gender governance, but also the gender attitudes that emerged during the conflict. In other words it seems that the cognitive space which developed as a result of the urgency of conflict and death allowed HIV to be considered as an issue which did not fit in that time and space. While at the same time, the same conditions created an environment that made many people vulnerable to HIV risks in their everyday lives.

The time line that is clearly articulated in the interviews shows the demo-bilization camps as the point at which they encountered HIV information at the end of the conflict. These camps are part of the overall international demobilization decommissioning reintegration (DDR) framework policies. The DDR process has become an important modality and a central part for many post-conflict peace-building interventions across the globe. The UN Secretary-General's Report on peacekeeping and DDR defines each compo-nent of the process as follows:

Disarmament
   is the collection of small arms and light and heavy weapons within a conflict zone. It frequently entails the assembly and cantonment of com-batants; it should also comprise the development of arms management programs, including their safe storage and their final disposition, which may entail their destruction. Demining may also be part of this process.
(UN 2000)

Demobilization
   refers to the process by which parties to a conflict begin to disband their military structures and combatants begin the transformation into civilian life. It generally entails registration of former combatants; some kind of assistance to enable them to meet their immediate basic needs; discharge, and transportation to their home communities. It may be fol-lowed by recruitment into a new, unified military force.

Reintegration
   refers to the process that allows ex-combatants and their families to adapt, economically and socially to productive civilian life. It generally entails provision of a package of cash or in-kind compensation, training and job- and income-generating projects
(UN S/2000/101)

In this structure the camps are threshold spaces delineating between the conflict and the post-conflict society as people, after being through the camps engage in reintegration processes within their own communities. It is in this context, that of creating civilians out of combatants, that the Burundian combatants going through the camps were also provided with HIV/AIDS-related information to sensitize them.

Changing lives, HIV/AIDS, and demobilization camps

The conflict in Burundi created many complex problems for those who were part of the conflict as combatants and for civilians who were exposed to the conflict due to their proximity to combatants and their social environment over the prolonged period of time. Given the length of time of the conflict social relations were altered. Different public spaces emerged. In many ways people were integrated into a public space shaped by fighting and the imminence of conflict. This integration to a public space created by the conflict alienated them from their normal social conditions. This alienation was partially underpinned by the cognitive distance from the everyday life they had before the conflict. This distancing was also exacerbated by sexual behavior in general and by the closely associated increase in sexual violence. Many felt, as mentioned by the group of ex-combatants in the first chapter, that these relations did not create the right kinds of conditions for life in the communities after the conflict. Many of these changed sexual relations had gendered implications, particularly for women who lived in the context of the conflict or near to combatants. The picture at the end of the conflict was bleak for many of these women who faced going back to their communities after becoming fighters, which indicated to people in their communities that these women had killed people. Furthermore, some men had to find a way of dealing with their bush wives and their children. Many male combatants also had to reflect on their own experiences of brutality in turn which had brutalized them. They realized there was a significant gap in social acceptability between the way they had lived during this period and the way they needed to live in their communities afterwards. Some of this realization surfaced as the end of the conflict approached, but most of it become apparent in demobilization camps that came with the DDR process in Burundi.

There are two questions about the end of the conflict that are important here. One of them is particularly relevant for the HIV/AIDS concerns: given the context that has been extensively discussed until now how far the DDR process, in particular its demobilization component in the camps, was able to engage with the vulnerabilities to HIV risks created during the conflict. The second question is about the DDR process: how far the DDR process was able to engage with these complex problems that were produced in the conflict. The next part of this chapter looks at the first question, while the conclusion provides a provisional answer to the second question, which will be tackled more broadly in Chapter 5.

As a prelude, this section provides a quick look at the DDR framework and its implementation in Burundi, but I am not going to rehearse the complex political and organizational mechanisms of the process extensively as there are in-depth studies which do this (Vrey and Boshoff 2006; Willems *et al.* 2010). The aim here is to consider the timeline of the DDR process and consider the way it was structured, together with the creation of a number of organizations to deal with it in Burundi by the international policy actors that were funding and facilitating the process. The way these actors developed policies and the organizational context of the implementation of these policies for DDR structured the outcomes for people who were exposed to them.

The Arusha Peace and Reconciliation Agreement for Burundi (The Arusha Accord) was signed on Monday August 28 2000, although the actual ceasefire and subsequent decrease in on-the-ground fighting in CNDD–FDD strongholds only took place when the CNDD–FDD agreed to sign a peace deal in November 2003. The Palipehutu–FNL remained outside of this until the May 2008 ceasefire. Alongside these, the African Union initially facilitated a disarmament, demobilization, and reintegration process. This was replaced in 2004 by a UN mission—the United Nations Operation in Burundi (ONUB). The Burundi DDR process was launched in December 2004 and closed in December 2008 with the completion of reinsertion processes. The second phase of the DDR dealings with the FNL began in 2009. Ex-combatants were processed in demobilization camps from December 2004 onwards and the first phase was nearly completed in September 2005 (Frey and Boshoff 2006: 9). The formal in-country program is funded by the World Bank Multi-country Demobilization and Reintegration Program (MDRP) and led by the national body *Commission National de Démobilisation, Réinsertion and Réintegration* (CNDRR). The Arusha agreement also required a number of other bodies to monitor the process such as The Implementation Monitoring Committee, which was responsible for implementation of the agreement, and The Joint Ceasefire Commission, which was to oversee the implementation of ceasefire agreements and the reform of the army.

One of the objectives of the DDR was to downsize the army to 25,000 and police to 15,000. All together, FAB and the rebel groups were estimated to have more than 55,000 troops. The DDR-based Joint Operations Plan (JOP) was issued on November 9 2004 (Frey and Boshoff 2005). The JOP set out a six-step procedure where ex-combatants were processed. There were two exit possibilities, with people either qualifying to join new armed forces or being demobilized as civilians. The JOP guideline set out a six-step process: "predisarmament assembly or cantonment; selection for demobilisation; disarmament of demobilising combatants; combatant status verification; demobilisation; and discharge" (Frey and Boshoff 2006: 26). By December 2008 a total of 23,022 adult ex-combatants were demobilized and received reinsertion support. In total 3,261 children were released from armed groups, 3,017 of whom received reinsertion support (MDRP 2009). Also according to an earlier report, 494 women had been demobilized (MDRP 2006). This number might have increased by 2008 but the above report does not mention numbers of women. Daley (2008) refers to 482 women being demobilized by May 2006 and Lemarchand (2009: 226) uses the number of 515 for women in his recent book. Daley (2008: 226) also shows that most of these women, 437, belonged to CNDD–FDD while FAB had no women demobilized from its ranks, although it had 2,273 children demobilized. In addition, at the end of the DDR program in "December 2008 18, 709 *Gardien de La Paix* and 9,674 *Militant Combatants* received one-time reinsertion payments" (MDRP 2009). The first group were militia armed by the government and collaborated with the army to protect neighborhoods and villages. Militant Combatants were similar groups armed by the rebels. Another group, the Civil Self-Defense Group (or "Civil self-defense in solidarity"), consisted of state employees receiving arms from the government to defend their neighborhoods (for a more extensive study on these group, see Pézard and Florquin 2007: 86–89).

The National DDR program policies only accepted those people as ex-combatants if they have been listed officially by the army (former FAB) and by the Burundian Armed Political Parties and Movements (APPM). Also, although many people were associated with fighting within the above-mentioned groups not all were officially considered ex-combatants in this initial criterion. This criterion was further elaborated as:

> A combatant will be defined as a person who served in armed conflict with at least one APPM or the FAB, and who was an active member of the fighting force of that movement before the signing of the Arusha Accord of 28 August 2000, the cease-fire agreement of 7 October 2002, the cease-fire agreement of 2 December 2002, and/or the cease-fire agreement of 16 November 2003.
>
> (UNDDR 2008)

This was an important reframing since it meant that the FAB and the APPM had to provide lists to verify people as their members in order for them to go through the DDR process. This was, of course, easier to demonstrate for those in the FAB, the regular army, than those in the APPM. In order to address this for the APPM it was established that an individual could "Testify his belonging to an APPM, being physically identified, registered on the legitimate authentic certified list submitted to the Joint Ceasefire Commission (JCC) and possess an individual weapon with munitions in a functional estate, or have access to a group weapon in accordance with the ratios specified in the annex to the present decree" or "Being recognized as combatant by the verification team in a Demobilization Center after having shown his military skills and having participated in military operations in Burundi or Democratic Republic of Congo with his APPM before the signature of the Ceasefire" (UNDDR 2008).

While it is important to have these criteria for operational reasons to facilitate the demobilization through the demobilization camps, it did not deal with a number of categories mentioned above, i.e., those self-demobilized individuals who quit the battlefield before cantonment and disarmament and were not recognized as ex-combatants. In contrast, most of these groups were recognized as ex-combatants in their own communities and also considered themselves a part of the conflict. Some, especially the *Gardien de La Paix*, have been claiming the reinsertion package since the very beginning of the DDR program since they threatened to derail the DDR process if they were not given resources, which led to the establishment of one-off reinsertion payments (Pézard and Florquin 2007). Another important issue particularly for our concerns is related to female combatants and those women and girls associated with fighting groups. Very few of the former were officially demobilized and the latter were not part of the process at all. There were many issues in relation to this situation. One was a function of the way the DDR system provided resources to allow people to reintegrate, in other words complete their cycle of becoming civilians once again (Coulter *et al.* 2008: 20–27).

Only officially demobilized ex-combatants, i.e., those with a demobilization card received in a demobilization camp were eligible for a cash reinsertion package. It was equivalent to an 18-month salary. The package was given in four parts. The first part was worth nine months' salary, given on exiting the demobilization camp. The following three parts were equal: each was worth three months' salary. The last three parts were delivered to the ex-combatant quarterly through the local bank network. When he/she left the demobilization camp, the ex-combatant was instructed to open a bank account on arrival in their region of origin. He/she would then go to the regional office of the SE/CNDRR to register and get bank ID registered so he/she could get the following payments. This also helped the SE/CNDRR know where ex-combatants were, at least during the 18-month period. When the DDR process was negotiated, it was decided that the calculation basis of the reinsertion would be the FAB-standard salary as of December 2002. The DDR was planned to start in 2003, but it was delayed until December 2004. The process was mandated by the UN Security Council resolution 1545 of May 21 2004. This salary standard differed depending on the rank of the soldier or officer. So, ex-combatants did not receive the same amount on demobilization camp exit and in the three subsequent payments. It was also agreed that rebel (CNDD–FDD) ranks would be recognized as equal to the ranks in the FAB. They called this *harmonization des grades*—harmonization of ranks.

This is the policy and organizational context within which combatants left their arms behind and were processed in demobilization camps. The above discussion of the details of the DDR process, point the way people were gradually impacted by the DDR process. By entering into the DDR process ex-combatants were entering into a set of new relations within a newly emerging institutional context that would regulate their lives as civilians. It is clear from the formation of the process that the sociability the camps provided was framed by needs of international security as mandated by the UN Security Council and the anxieties of the newly emerging political authority in the country. In this manner, the DDR process presented an important opportunity to deal with the problems created and experienced by many during the conflict. The nature of gender relations that emerged during the conflict and HIV presented important constraints for reintegration and living in the communities. Thus, it is critical to consider whether the DDR process managed to engage with these problems. This analysis provides a way of understanding the complexity in the post-conflict context and emerging vulnerabilities to HIV.

In his reflections "I" discussed his experience in the demobilization camp and what he thought of being told about HIV/AIDS at the time.

I: It was useful to be told. Useful for me because they advised to test in the camp. They also advised wives to be tested. At some point when I came home I got tested, a second time with my wife before having sex with her because I am respectful. I had suspicions of HIV/AIDS because in 1998 I spent three days with a girl, she was studying, and also after that I had sex with someone else. So I was not comfortable, I thought I could be HIV+ I suspected me, not my wife.

INTERVIEWER: So you had your first test in the camp?

I: Yes.

INTERVIEWER: How did it take place?

I: You go into the place they are testing, they will not register you, they ask you why you want to be tested you tell them because you want to know your status. If healthy, or not, you know how to behave in the future. So if HIV+ you know how to treat yourself and behave, if negative you know how to protect and not go into HIV risk. They told me to return the next morning, then the doctor asked me how would I react if I were ill. I said that if I were HIV+ I will accept it for what things are and it was God who planned it for me. He told me that I was healthy – that my blood was fine. In my heart it was not easy, I was troubled. It was like I wish not to be in front of that doctor, it was difficult. I thought if I am HIV+ I might not be alone, there were others, I must accept because I cannot change it. I lived there [in the camp] for two weeks at the time I was tested. Since the beginning I had seen images on TV. There was a facilitator who told us to test, they did not force us to do it. I think only 10 percent of people went to test. People asked—how was it like? People would say they take large quantities of blood you will suffer. In reality they took very small amount, some went after that. Some said you only go if you think you are HIV+, me I am healthy I don't need to go. You could have gone to test when you wanted. Few went at the beginning, towards the middle after some had HIV results it encouraged others to go.

INTERVIEWER: How was the HIV/AIDS training?

I: It was on Monday, Wednesday and Thursday—three days, two hours each day. It was mandatory. You had to be in the place except for those who were ill. Some listened to the discussion and it went to their hearts. Others just said that this guy [facilitator] is here only to make money, others did not say much. For most it was difficult, they did not understand the information.

INTERVIEWER: Why?

I: We really heard the message but really did not think about HIV/AIDS information at that moment, we thought about the life after the camp—when money was not coming. If I could I would choose a moment when people are likely to listen—may be after people received their money [reinsertion package] and were more likely to listen.

The process and the environment within which HIV/AIDS interventions were introduced to ex-combatants present some important issues. The psychology of the ex-combatants appears to be a confounding factor for impacting their lives in relation to HIV. Furthermore, given the experiences of people and the nature of the HIV information, the timing of such interventions is called into question. I's reflections on why some resisted testing in the camp paint a picture of the difficulty to engage with the discourse on HIV. The discourse might ignite someone's sense of being combatant. It challenges the perspective developed in the conflict, that of being a combatant, with another that is essentially based on being ill with HIV. Furthermore, in this swap the latter position associates the person in the camp with sexual activity in the context of the conflict. This had significant implications for the person in terms of reintegration as mentioned in the first chapter in many of the discussions with the ex-combatants.

These issues were further unpicked in the reflections of J when he talked about his experiences in the camp.

J: From joining to the war until leaving it I never talked about HIV/AIDS. We had this training only one week in the camp. We learned a lot on how to live with community and things on HIV/AIDS. All these things were done very quickly; all were very fast and superficial.

INTERVIEWER: Were people perceptive in these sessions?

J: Really we were not focused. Some even skipped these and went to have beer outside. Anyway, it could have been more useful. It would have been more useful to have these discussions and the information on HIV/AIDS in community and with other people. For us the week was long as we wanted to go home, but it was too short for really learning new things, learning was too superficial. It would have been better to have this with others. This could help decrease discrimination and would help reintegration. There would be more time and opportunity to really understand things.

INTERVIEWER: Were you tested?

J: In the demobilization camp they tested us. May be it was compulsory. … it was not, but kind of, it was highly encouraged. They had a strategy: they advised us to go to this person to see if we had any problems/disabilities in order to be helped when we are back at home. And they tested us for HIV among other things. They gave us the results the last day just before we left the camp. That day, it was difficult to know and share ideas with others. They planned the testing results to be given at the last moment. You went to the office and at the last minute you went into the office to get HIV results. If you were found HIV—you were pleased and thought of being careful and abstinent. If not, you knew you should use condom. We had already been told that one has been lucky not to die in the war and to be careful. After the HIV results you went straight on to the bus.

INTERVIEWER: Was there any counseling?

J: We were in a hurry to go home. One could say I am healthy while going to the bus. People went out fast one after the other. We had no time to talk to each other. On the bus we did not talk about HIV. Really we did not talk about the past (HIV was part of the past) we talked about the future; what we will do when we arrive at home. We were very anxious about our future, of the next steps, not about our past.

Here J is reiterating, like "I," the mindset of many ex-combatants in the demobilization camps. The combination of the limited time to be processed in the camps and the wish to have time to adjust were creating barriers to engage with the information on HIV. From the perspective of the people who facilitated these processes, some of these issues were also frustrating. One senior reintegration expert, while talking about the need to give more information to ex-combatants, reflected on her experience with the demobilization camps.

Some information is not well understood by people. There are some misinterpretations. Ex-combatants spent approximately two weeks in the demobilization camps. In this the time was not enough to get all the necessary information. Sometimes, the ex-combatants themselves were asking for more information. When they were in the Demobilization Camp, ex-combatants were not clearly aware of the HIV testing. Many were tested without knowing they were being tested. You know, there were more than 500 people in each camp. They were in such a state of mind that they did not pay attention. For example former FAB soldiers were uncomfortable as they knew they just lost their jobs. They were anxious about the immediate future.

This reflection focuses on the issue of the importance of the mind and the awareness of those going through a process. In terms of HIV it is interesting to reflect that many were aware of testing, but may not have been fully clear of the implications of testing. The context within which the testing process took place also seems to have had an effect on people's behavior. According to Q, a facilitator who worked in three demobilization camps on HIV sensitization, the ex-combatants were approached through indirect methods.

Q: In a standard program in these camps there were usually two people on the stage may be a singer and actor who worked the room. Initially there was also one facilitator but then there were two. At times there also was a theatre troupe. They played scenes relevant to HIV stereotypes for instance on soldiers and prostitutes. Facilitators had the central role while other singing and acting facilitators raised questions and answered those raised by the ex-combatants. They talked about modes of transmission, how to prevent and other relevant issues. Ex-combatants usually said that they did not know, in the bush we were kind of already dead, if not from HIV, then from a bullet. There were stories of rape, sometimes of one woman by many men. Facilitators tried correct miss-understandings about sharing a house, toilet or eating together and hand-shakes. We told ex-combatants that with saliva, the risk was very weak, you need liters of saliva. We also gave advice on testing. If we knew people who were tested negative we congratulated them and then pushed for behavior change. If we knew they were HIV+ we told them it was better to know and we advised them to stop drinking alcohol, stop doing hard work and avoid much sexual activity. We advised them to use condom always even if they are married.

When they arrived most of them knew nearly nothing. For former rebels they had never heard of HIV. It was the first time for them. When we asked what they already knew about HIV/AIDS response were often "we had no time for that," "we sometimes heard about something on the radio," "four years ago we had sex with one woman and she is dead now" and some were very surprised by it. For FAB they did know something. Out of the training room some ex-combatants talked about rape. Some said that their commanders were severe on sexual relations that there were serious punishments even if the relationships were consensual.

INTERVIEWER: Do you think ex-combatants benefited from this process?

Q: People were just coming out of the bush and from fighting. They were not in the mood of learning. We needed to progressively create an environment, with plays, songs and jokes. Sometimes they had no reaction. They began clapping in rhythm with traditional songs, and we included "ice-breakers." Our animation style was very dynamic and participatory, so they progressively opened up. Sometimes some participants thanked us for having talked to them about HIV/AIDS. Some others were saying "No, I don't want testing. I would be depressed and may commit suicide." They were anxious about their future.

We had a play showing both low-ranked soldiers and high-ranking officers competing for the same woman. Then when describing themselves in the play, they used the expression "Abasubijwe mu buzima budasanzwe—those who have been put into non-usual (not normal) life." Ex-combatants used half-jokingly this expression to refer to their status in the demobilization camp and outside. The official statement in talking about ex-combatants refers to "Abasubijwe mu buzima busanzwe"—those who have been put back into normal life. Ex-combatants were also more direct and cared less about taboo and were less constrained. They asked really crude questions and were more out-spoken than civilians. Civilians show more social, cultural constraints when speaking. They would not ask direct questions.

INTERVIEWER: Were there women ex-combatants?

Q: There were no women among FAB. There were in rebel groups. They had questions like shall we give orders to our husbands? If our husbands are with other women what do we do? Both men and women had similar difficulties to understand and asked similar questions. They did not directly talk about rape … they implied things. They said, for instance that a woman was abducted and brought into the bush. After two weeks she said "I prefer to stay here." I think very few women volunteered.

INTERVIEWER: Did they talk about implications of being HIV+?

Q: Many were afraid. This idea was frozen in their heads. They said that being positive was a punishment from God. It is unthinkable for them as "normal" human beings. Some young men would say "if I found my wife is HIV+ I flee from her, I chase her away or I would kill her"; "it is not good to live with someone who is HIV+. We need God to put clear signs on their faces so we could avoid them" or "we should not go to toilet after an HIV+ person" and wanted to separate people with HIV+ from their own eating areas. As a result no HIV+ person could talk about it. I saw one person. He almost killed himself. He was mad after he knew he was HIV+. He was emotionally very affected. Also some came to me after our sessions personally to talk about their personal issues. They usually ask about how to live with HIV and say "I was found with AIDS," "I was told that I have the HIV virus when and how shall I get medication." But no one declared clearly and thoughtfully their status.

INTERVIEWER: When would it have been better to train people for HIV/AIDS?

Q: I think the best moment should have been before they arrived in the camps. The training could have used a command structure since as combatants they were used to obey orders. Our training was in all a day or half a day. It was not enough. There should have been more time so we could have split them into small groups and had a more interactive process. We really needed more time to enrich their knowledge. Our terms of reference had narrowed the scope of sensitization. To achieve a real behavior change we needed much more than what was planned.

I don't understand for instance why follow-up sessions to be held in their communities were not more planned. Ex-combatants needed to be trained within their own communities and with their neighbors. This could have also helped us to monitor the impact of the first training and to shape a complementary training based on how ex-combatants were reacting to real life.

Most of these reflections paint a picture in which people entered the demobilization camps and were processed through a set of training programs and then sent off to their communities for reintegration. Furthermore, the sociability in these camps was clearly inhibiting since many people were meeting each other for the first time outside of the conflict, creating anxieties about a kind of civilian normality. This was not conducive for dealing with the problems ex-combatants were facing at the end of the long conflict.

As a part of this process, if one considers the problems that have been highlighted so far in relation to gender relations and HIV the circumstances in the camps were inadequate to deal with many of these issues. In terms of gender relations, mostly absent female combatants and other women from the process did not allow proper engagement with what had happened in the conflict in relation to gender relations. Furthermore, Q's reflection on the answers he had from ex-combatants points out that some men, when introduced to HIV information, attributed the problem to women and considered HIV their fault. In this they were not reflecting on their own role in creating the conditions for vulnerability to HIV and catching HIV. During the conflict traditional gender norms had been stretched to their limits, instrumentalizing women; at the end of the conflict once the HIV question surfaced for many ex-combatants, women were then held responsible for the problem.

A further challenging issue is the realization of how significant this HIV problem might be for ex-combatants after not thinking about it or not realizing its existence during the conflict. The time component here is important. The pace of training and testing in the camps were part of the demobilization process. The HIV/AIDS component of this process involved group sensitization. While this might be a good start considering the context out of which ex-combatants were coming, it did not encourage the right way of engaging with the discussion. The reaction from many ex-combatants was to take a position linked to the masculine outlook they had developed in the conflict. It seems that the logic of the process was driven by the need for a rapid processing of people back into civilian life. This logic did not consider the psycho-social needs of ex-combatants in terms of how to engage with HIV, which was necessary for behavior change and which ultimately was about how to engage with their gender perceptions. The issue was treated as a technical intervention within a package that needed to be delivered, and at the end of the course it was assumed that ex-combatants were sensitized in a functional manner that would change their behavior. However, given their state of mind the link from sensitization to behavior change might be a complex process with repeated interventions. According to a specialist on social integration and gender in Bujumbura:

> Gender issues were not focused by CNDRR. Activities were planned for sensitizing ex-combatants on STI and gender. This was in the initial work plan. Some things were done for sensitization on STI and HIV/AIDS when ex-combatants were in demobilization camps. But nothing has been done on the gender theme.

Conclusion

The conflict created an information vacuum on HIV as a concern for people's behavior. The knowledge that pre-dated 1993 gradually disappeared in this vacuum. Many ex-combatants, particularly the young who joined the rebellion, did not consider HIV as an issue. For those old enough to be exposed to HIV information before 1993, the nature of the conflict and the imminence of fighting changed their order of priorities. This also led to a gradual disappearance of discussions on HIV/AIDS. The gender governance discussed in the earlier chapters made it impossible for women to engage in discussion of sexually transmitted infections (STIs) or HIV. At the same time, the conflict conditions made many women more and more exposed to these problems. The training provided on HIV and STIs in the demobilization camps as a part of DDR intervened in this challenging psychological and social context. People were trying to adjust to changing circumstances at multiple levels. I argue above that the demobilization component of the DDR process in the demobilization camps was insensitive to gender vulnerabilities—both to those that frame the social relations in Burundi and to those that were created during the conflict. As pointed out earlier in the chapter, the selection criteria established for demobilization already created a problem which is also clearly indicated by the numbers of people who were demobilized. Those women who were part of the conflict in various ways as fighters, camp followers, or in some kind of support role to the fighters were discounted from the process as a matter of structure. A further complication was the requirement for APPM groups to provide combatants lists for these people to be included in the DDR process. There were very significant problems with this approach. In short, the DDR process did not deal with so called *self-demobilized*.

The conditions under which women in particular became self-demobilized is also important to understand (also see McKay and Mazurana 2004). Considering the way women were treated by the rebel groups during the conflict, it seems unlikely that group leaderships would have supported women to go through a formal process. One aspect of this is the resources that were made available for ex-combatants through the formal process. Here the oversight, discussed in the literature, that considers women and young women in these contexts not as combatants but as "camp followers" might have been tactically deployed (Fox 2004: 469; also see Brett 2004), particularly given that the gender component of the National DDR program states that men and women have to be treated equally and to receive the same package and services. Considering the above exclusions, this equal treatment clearly remained unrealized. It was only possible if women went into the camps. Although there is an official DDR gender coordinator and program, few resources and tangible policies were implemented toward gender issues. Women's associations, for instance, complained that there were no specific indicators in DDR for reintegration of female ex-combatants, even if they had been through the camps.

Another aspect is related to the sexual violence and abuse that might have become an issue if the women were demobilized in formal processes. Furthermore, as highlighted by Mary-Jane Fox young women's experiences created "an affront to and a major departure from established norms" (2004:

466). The processes of going into the camps deterred a lot of women who were fighters. As a result, the DDR immediately created a gendered problem, as many women affected by the conflict remained outside the DDR process. Many women, and low-ranking men, were not listed in these declarations by their commanders. They were simply sent directly back to their communities. Given the gender dynamics between women and ranking rebels, it would have been very difficult to resist this coercive support for women to self-demobilize. In other words, right at the end of the conflict gender governance was instrumental in disenfranchising women once again. Some were sent away because they were pregnant or with young children, under the pretext of it would be better for them to be in their own homes. In this way, many bush wives were reportedly prevented from receiving DDR benefits. It was also pointed out in the interviews that ranked rebels did not want their bush wives to claim married status in the camps as many of them maintained families in their own communities too.

On the whole, the complications created by the DDR are obvious if one considers the process and its aims in relation to the dynamics and compli- cated relations of the conflict: the DDR process tries to forge a new army by on the one hand reducing the number of people who had taken up arms; on the other hand it addressed security sector concerns after the conflict. At the same time, it was an attempt for the APPM to transform themselves into political parties without armed groups being attached to them. This was an essential part of the transition to an electoral system. As a result, they focused on a very limited number of people. For instance, Daley argues that the:

> DDR appears to reward militarism and has had limited success because of its financial inducements have been small. Rather than the state re- establishing its monopoly on violence, DDR under neo-liberalism seems to spawn more privatized and atomized forms of militarism.
>
> (Daley 2008: 35)

While this might be true in some contexts, it seems that in Burundi the DDR program was also built to consolidate the power of the emerging political authority and to allow them more negotiation space. This is even more the case if we consider the situation from the gender perspective. The process allowed the emerging leadership to entirely ignore the gendered outcomes of the conflict and their role in creating some of the circumstances women found themselves in during the conflict. It also allowed them subsequently to side- line the implications of women's experiences in creating particular social and material needs. This had much broader social implications, as the absence of gender concerns closed down any space to negotiate and push for a change in the gender relations on the basis of the experiences from the conflict. Those experiences disappeared from the discussion as socio-political needs to be addressed. This was also a process in which the reintegration payment at least for the rebels meant that the APPPM leadership appeared to deliver resources to their followers and in this way they also unburdened themselves from responsibility to deliver broader social integration resources into their communities.

While talking about the emerging political power and its machinations, it is important not to lose sight of the influence of international policy process. The DDR process was framed and supported by international actors, mostly by the World Bank with support from various countries. The discussions above show that this international policy approach was broadly gender blind. This was mostly due to their concerns that were based on understanding of what amounts to security in the region and how they could make sure that it is established. The stability of the emerging power dynamics was more important for their concerns. It seems for these reasons they expediently did not pay too much attention to the people's experiences in their attempts to create mechanisms leading to a more stable Burundi.

Considered from gender and HIV perspectives, the DDR process represents a missed opportunity. Rather than acting as a "transformative social space" to allow people to engage with their experiences (Campbell and Cornish 2010: 1573), the process was framed within a limited scope focused on state security. As important as this may be, this focus did not allow the creation of attitudes to influence peoples' behavior that had implications for many communities. I agree with one of the main conclusions by Willems *et al.* that "Looking at how DDR has been perceived on the ground, one must conclude DDR in Burundi has not been successful in terms of economic reintegration" (2010: 3). One of the reasons for this remains the gender governance which underwrites socio-economic relations after the conflict. They remained untouched by the process discussed here. The DDR created further complications in terms of integration and addressing people's social needs, including the ones on HIV/AIDS created by the conflict. From the HIV/AIDS perspective the DDR was also a missed opportunity as its concerns framed the target groups for limited outcomes in relation to a perception of security.

5 Discontent with reintegration

Once ex-combatants leave demobilization camps they begin a new phase of the DDR process—reintegration. This chapter will look at the experiences of ex-combatants in this process and the challenges faced by both ex-combatants and their communities. The idea of reintegration assumes that people are returning to their own communities and they need to socialize within the community to become a part of it once more. The implicit idea is that these ex-combatants have severed relations with their communities. Here, the idea of reintegration needs to be considered as a two-way process: it is not only about the ex-combatants' aim to become a part of their community but it is also about the communities' assessment of how far they would like to engage with these ex-combatants. In other words, it is a process in which communities assess their relationship with those coming back after the conflict. At a micro-level, it is also about reintegration within families.

The formal reintegration process was linked to the DDR and resources attached to it. There were also thousands of so called "self-demobilized" people, including large numbers of women, who did not benefit from these resources. The reintegration was experienced differently at various levels depending on the exit routes taken from the conflict. The gender differences in combination with these exit routes also created variations in people's experiences of reintegration. The formal route created its own problems. During the demobilization camp process each ex-combatant was asked to choose his preferred reintegration option out of five: (i) formal education (going back to school), (ii) entrepreneurship (expanding an existing business), (iii) vocational skills training (car driving, computer literacy, etc.), (iv) employment (former civil servants going back to government paid jobs), and (v) income-generating activities. While people went through demobilization camps, they did not have material or social resources to engage with reintegration. The opportunity to have the reintegration package on return to their community was also an important way to negotiate acceptance into the community for many male ex-combatants. It would have meant creating a small business or having more resources than others in the community, thus allowing them to be accepted. However, in practice things turned out differently.

The formal process also created complications for those who were expecting a resources package to help engage with their community. The last cycle of delivery of this integration package, described in the last chapter, was still under way in May 2008. It meant that some ex-combatants who were receiving the package had waited nearly three years to have access to this funding. There was a gap between leaving the camps as a demobilized person and having access to the resources that would facilitate their reintegration. This created particularly difficult circumstances for younger ex-combatants who were not married or without families. It made it difficult for them to go back to their community as ex-combatants without resources. Even for those who had families it was an embarrassing situation to return to the community without resources. This then led to a situation where ex-combatants stayed as groups in urban areas, particularly in Bujumbura. They were trying to agitate, as discussed in the introduction, to expedite the situation. The lack of resources and employment created an unstable and volatile environment in these locations. The lack of resources and the prolonged delay in the distribution of the reintegration package meant that a further social stigma developed in relation to ex-combatants, hindering their reintegration. This was also not a gender-blind process. For women combatants it was even worse, as many were not part of this demobilization process and they had to find other means to survive. One such means was sex-work, or transactional sex, which was for some the only available option. Male ex-combatants staying in urban spaces for longer periods and drinking also created the context for sex-work. This on the whole had a further impact on the way communities considered these groups and their reintegration within their social contexts. Another issue at the end of the conflict and reintegration process was long-term refugees returning from Tanzania after years of living in refugee camps. Many of these people were long-term refugees who had left the country in the 1970s. Their return was complicated by the land questions. Those who had owned land were now hoping to claim it back. As a result, their return also complicated the resource questions.

T began by talking about her job and her experiences as one of the social reintegration specialists in the formal process managed under CNDRR.

T: I work on the social integration of ex-combatants into their communities of origin. There are many ex-combatants who come to demand say "I have HIV." They come to me asking for medicines and for food support. But the CNDRR program has not planned such a thing to support ex-combatants living with HIV. I sent them to NGOs, to associations that could help them with treatment and support. During the war, in the bush, sexual contact was easy and frequent. Mainly women were sexually taken by force. In the bush, people had no time to think about HIV. But after demobilization we saw that there were HIV+ ex-combatants who needed special support. I have personally seen many HIV+ ex-combatants who came to me looking for support. They are afraid of AIDS, they also care not to infect others, and also want to keep their lives as long as possible to help their families. Some regret not having money and also worry about the efforts families are putting to keep them. They see that they cannot help their families that much. Some people complained that they were stigmatized by their community, especially about being slim and having colored spots on their skins. We encouraged ex-combatants to go for voluntary testing so they would know their status and have the appropriate behavior. I did not see personally many ex-combatants asking for testing after the demobilization camps in the community. Not all ex-combatants came back for their results.

We have mixed-associations of ex-combatants. For example, I visited recently a women-ex-combatant association in Mutimbuzi commune. They planted cassava and other plants. Those women talked about many problems. One of those problems is that there is no HIV/AIDS component of our program (CNDRR's reintegration program). Those women were tested when they were in the Demobilization Camp. They did not go back to take their results. So they don't know their status. Those women are taking care of orphans and some of those children are orphaned because of AIDS. Association members receive information on HIV/AIDS from other partners [NGOs].

INTERVIEWER: How did their experiences in the conflict impact their reintegration?

T: Women were abducted by fighters and became either combatants' wives, combatants, or they were sort of laborers for fighters. Often they were sexually abused by different men in the bush. The risks were high. Many women went to the bush alone. They usually are not comfortable to talk about this subject. They complain often that their husbands did not accept them when they came back. This subject is hard to talk as it is very emotional. They should be helped to have a space to express their feelings. This could help them to open up to themselves. Ex-combatants were interested in HIV/AIDS information in demobilization camps as it was about prevention. We did an evaluation and they said that they were happy with the training. They said that the training was too short and expressed their need for more training. So I would say it was a good start for them.

INTERVIEWER: What are the main problems for integration?

T: The fundamental problem is social stigmatization as some ex-combatants tend to be rejected by their communities. People say they are killers and they are being awarded through the DDR program. We see this on the ground. We work in collaboration with the local administration in order to have the community accept ex-combatants. Usually, for instance, there are many instances of theft. People say that ex-combatants are responsible, even when no one is caught. There is a lot of suspicion. Ex-combatants have economic and financial problems, as they lost employment, salaries and some lost land. Some of them are really needy.

It is also very hard for young women ex-combatants. Most of them are not married. It is difficult for them as they are seen as they were "bush wives" for male combatants. No man in the community wants to marry them. Young male combatants are in a better situation when they have some resources. They have no problem in finding someone to marry. What people ask them is to have land, resources and money. You know the reinsertion package is enough money in the view of community members. Former FAB soldiers find it very difficult to manage the reinsertion package, as they find it a small amount, not enough to meet their needs. If a young FAB soldier is demobilized before having his house built and getting married the life becomes difficult. When an ex-combatant spent his reinsertion package well by making some small investment, and starting some income generating activity, he tends to succeed in his business.

INTERVIEWER: Are you able to follow how re-insertion packages are used?

T: The follow up on ex-combatant micro-projects is done by implementation partners. This is useful for ex-combatant business development. Also we have Provincial Offices [Bureau Provincial] in which we have staff responsible for helping ex-combatants to have information and guidance. In the offices there is a responsible officer (Responsible du Bureau Provincial and an assistant *Assistant chargé du Suivi Evaluation*). In terms of HIV/AIDS political leaders have strongly asserted their will to deal with the problem. They created a ministry to fight HIV/AIDS.

There are still lots to be done to sensitize ex-combatants on HIV/AIDS. Ex-combatants don't know much and they arrive in a community which is also not very informed or has no information at all. This makes an ex-combatant's life difficult. It would have been better if they had arrived in well sensitized communities. Even here in the town in some quarters there are people who are not very careful about HIV.

In the communities people don't think too much about the HIV aspect of the situation. What make people fear and wonder is ex-combatants' violent past. They are fearful of what these people were doing in the past: killing and stealing. The biggest fear is related with theft and killings. There is no fear related with HIV/AIDS specifically among ex-combatants. In the community, there are many different people with HIV so there is no specific concern about ex-combatants. About rape this phenomenon is not associated with ex-combatants in the community perception. Ex-combatants are not much accused of rape in the community. It is said that when rape happens (now) ex-combatants might be as guilty as much as anyone else. The most expressed fear is not about HIV, it is about violence in the community. Also, ex-combatants are a small percentage of the population in each community. In some areas, such as Bujumbura Rural, some ex-combatants fear violence that could come from the FNL fighters [at the time of these interviews FNL was still fighting outside Bujumbura in the Bujumbura Rural]. Some prefer to quit their communities and want to reintegrate in Bujumbura town. Some ex-combatants fear revenge attacks as they committed many crimes during the war. This seems to happen to some ex-combatants so you could find some ex-combatants from Makamba trying to reintegrate in Kirundo or Ruyigi. Most of those changing locations prefer towns as they are looking for more work opportunities.

T's reflections not only provide insights on the way reintegration was planned and the way people experienced the process but also how this process was about transforming combatant subjectivities into civilian subjectivities that are compatible with community perspectives. Here the hyper-masculinity that emerged during the conflict created problems for many male ex-combatants. Furthermore, it is important to reflect on some of her points in the light of her governmental position in the CNDRR. It is clear that within the DDR process, overseen by CNDRR, HIV was not a central concern. This is also evident in the way the DDR process was framed in a very limited manner. Once ex-combatants were processed and received their reinsertion package they became civilians. As a result their particular needs, which could be defined broadly as wellbeing concerns due to their economic and health conditions, were not part of the policy concerns for actors dealing with DDR. If we consider this from the HIV perspective, the issue is rather dramatic as it is clear that although during the camps ex-combatants were given basic understanding of HIV and some were tested, on the whole the intervention at that moment did not create a significant impact on behavior. Also the delay in the distribution of resources from the DDR process led to a concentration of poor and stigmatized ex-combatants living in towns. These circumstances created further vulnerabilities to HIV risks, and the DDR process did not have any means to deal with this situation which was the function of its own delivery. Even if T is indicating that ex-combatants were satisfied with the HIV training, the way she then talks about them being more demanding for HIV information and training suggests that ex-combatants were questioning the continuity of the intervention.

Here there is also an underlying process with regards to the relationship between the rebel ex-combatants and the new political authority that had relied on many of these ex-combatants in its struggle to achieve its aims over a long period of time. The DDR process allowed ex-combatants to be significantly distanced from the political authority and it resource relations. The insertion package is seen by some, as discussed in the introduction, as a payback to ex-combatants delivering on the promises of resources they were given during the conflict. At the same time, their well-being needs linked to being ex-combatants were ignored. Some of these needs clearly manifested themselves once these ex-combatants became civilians and, therefore, they were outside the purview of the military resource distribution system. They were not going to have any entitlements to welfare resources on education, health, or employment on the basis of being veterans. It appeared that the political authority has passed the responsibility of engaging with ex-combatants and delivery of services on these issues to other groups, those that were not part of the political discussion such as local associations, local NGOs, and international NGOs.

This was not just a resource problem. It was also an important psychological issue as the combatants had enjoyed power which had developed into a particular kind of hyper-masculinity during the conflict. It was through this masculinity and its performance that they established their social relations and engagement within communities during the conflict. Not all combatants, as the discussion in Chapter 2 shows, agreed with this masculinity. However, all acted according to its boundaries at various points to be included and to survive. As a result, they benefitted from the patriarchal dividend established in this context. The dividend facilitated the instrumentalization of women as a resource for the cause and allowed some combatants to survive while also maintaining ranked officers' power and control. This gendered process no doubt created an important power imbalance in the way combatants considered themselves and their relationship with the communities. Arguably, some justified their abusive relationship either with women or other men who were not within their groups on the basis of being part of the larger patriarchal context. At the end of the demobilization for ex-combatants, their social environment and the patriarchal norms that regulated that context disappeared. They found themselves in an altered gendered context from the one which produced and reproduced their hyper-masculinity. Furthermore, this context required them to understand the consequences of their actions. Once they were back in the community, their past was now re-evaluated from a different register in the community.

The point raised by T in relation to the stigmatization of ex-combatants as killers is an important issue that challenges the gender identity they formed during the conflict. The fact that their ranking officers also seemed to let them go with little resources pointed to another level of problems with their psychology. The implications of all these issues were also very significant for women. Issues were more complicated for them as many were also partnered with combatants and had had children during the conflict. Therefore, the stigma towards returning women was not only focused on them being *killers*, but more on them being used by many men in the bush. The source of this view is undoubtedly linked to the way the gender governance situates women in Burundi. T reflects on the fact that many of these women, also many men, did not have any space or forum to discuss or come to terms with what happened to them during the conflict. Many interviewees also discussed this issue, i.e., that no one had asked them about their experiences and that many just wanted them to disappear once they had finished the DDR process. However, this also raises the question of why CNDRR was not interested in this discussion and did not create space for this kind of engagement with the ex-combatants.

One probable answer is the political stakes that this kind of discussion would have created for the new political authority. Many women were abducted and exposed to different kinds of abuse and many of them were from those communities associated with rebels. This suggests that women talking about their experiences after the end of the conflict would have been at best embarrassing and at worst raise criminal questions for some of the ex-rebel officers who had now become politicians. Another aspect of this was raised by T when she talked about the way communities think about rape when it happens. She pointed out clearly that ex-combatants were not directly accused. When there is no space to talk about the past silence allowed women to function better in their communities since talking about being abused or raped will not help them. Silence also works for ex-combatants not to face questions about these issues. In other words, the gender imbalances and the way they influenced resource allocation in the communities maintained women's silences on these issues.

On the whole, in the reintegration process ex-combatants inevitably became part of the memory of violence. In order to break from this memory they had to contribute to their communities in different ways and perform a role which breaks away from their identification with the conflict. HIV/AIDS become challenging at this juncture, as indicated by A earlier in the interviews. The possibility of testing, and testing HIV+, would signify a constant link with their past during the conflict. This would unravel their attempts to construct non-conflict masculine subjectivities within Burundian gender governance. Such a link with the past and the status of HIV+ would challenge their status within their communities, as sexual abuse and violence remain unacceptable within those communities. Furthermore, it would also question their future contributions to those communities. These considerations create impediments for engaging with HIV discourse. This difficult situation adds further to the vulnerabilities created to HIV risks after the conflict, as a result of the events during the conflict.

Two ex-combatants, U who was 24 and V who was 40 at the time of the interview, were involved in the reintegration process in Nyanza. They were talking about the difficulties of the process.

U: Reintegration was and is hard, sometimes I wish I could fly away to somewhere where no one knows I am an ex-combatant. People blame stealing on ex-combatants, if you are in business and you do well, people wonder how you are doing well. I have a business, but it is hard still authorities in my hillside think that I am bad. We even collected small arms to improve our image, but it did not work. People said that the arms were just part of what is there, that we stole the rest or we just disarm only people from certain political party and not others. I wish to return to FDN [newly formed army] I would give my demob package back, and return to the army if they give me the opportunity.

When an ex-combatant and local girl gets together, her family pushes him away because of ex-combatant image. It happened to my friends and to me personally four times. Some have not succeeded to marry yet, this increase the HIV as they are having sex with many people. Let me explain better. Before, during the war, the soldiers [FAB] posted here for protection a soldier will take a wife in the commune, then drop her when he left and he would take another wherever he goes. This increased the wrong image of soldiers and for us too, as we were soldiers too. People saw soldiers as man who could not keep his wife. Another thing is that rebels are seen as bad as those who hurt people.

v: People think that we stole things because we have money. Even the administration believed theft was caused by ex-combatants. If we say in a meeting we were disarmed, many don't believe us. We asked people to name the thief individually to see whether he was really an ex-combatant. People forget there were wrong doers in the normal population. We also had disadvantage: for example some NGOs build houses for people but they refuse to help us to build house they say ex-combatants had funds from CNDRR. Some thought that ex-combatants were rich. In some cases they give resources to people and then when they realized these are ex-combatants they want to take those back. Another case was in Kabonga, an NGO gave some resources to people and then "told" that these were ex-combatants and they took the items back. But these were not ex-combatants.

   When these kinds of things happen we feel bad. CNDRR say we are like others in the community but we are not treated as such. For example, I have heard three ex-combatants were refused marriage because of who they are. The decision rests with the father.

INTERVIEWER: What would help ex-combatants?

u: Jobs, this would help our image it would give us means doing agriculture. Now people laugh at us they say so you have been demoted. We need to develop our leadership skills it will help in the future it will help us to speak when we are pushed aside. People don't include us in things like trainings. I was trained as a car mechanic but employers hate us they would rather train a new person than hire me who is already trained. We need the state's support to be accepted we need jobs so we are not the poorest in the community. We can do many jobs we can do many things other than shoot guns. We just want opportunity so we are accepted and our bad image can be removed.

The discussion highlights some of the difficulties that are experienced by ex-combatants in the reintegration process. The determining factor here is the attitudes of the community towards ex-combatants. Note that the mockery reported about being demoted shows that the community is not intimidated by ex-combatants, but is in fact intimidating them by bringing up their changed circumstances since the end of the conflict. This undoubtedly creates an exclusionary cycle at many levels for ex-combatants, one which might underwrite the reaction of those fathers who reject relations between their daughters and ex-combatants.

   There were of course exceptions. According to a local observer and reintegration specialist:

   the nature of reintegration was also influenced by the politics too. Some of the young ex-combatants from the bush are linked with the government. They become influential in the community level where CNDD–FDD is in power.

They identify three important implications of the negative attitudes they have experienced in creating instability in their lives. The first is the difficulty in getting married, the second is establishing a kind of economic stability to maintain their lives, and the last one is the more generalized issue of constant suspicion which determines their activities within the community. In one of the interviews an ex-combatant was very clear when he said that:

> We were supported, but with a small package—when fighting we hurried to destroy and now we are back and all is destroyed and we need start-up support. I wish the World Bank would give more support, not money, but training, information in woodworking, for instance, could help. Money does not help us to learn a living.

In these circumstances, women's situation was even more tenuous. Most were self-demobilized and their experiences in the bush located them outside the expected gender behavior in their communities. No one questioned the fact that the same gender governance made them exposed and vulnerable during the conflict. In an interview with the students who joined the rebellion, they talked about their lives in the bush and how difficult it was, as reported in chapter 3. Their views on the reintegration process were also revealing. The first view expressed by W implicitly compared their life after the conflict to their life in the bush. She said that *No problems, we are used to tough life. Now we are trying to establish ourselves in a neighborhood.* X on the other hand was more explicit:

> Of course there are problems in coming back. You have a child and not enough money. Combatants are not received well. If there is an attack ex-combatants are accused. They see us as bad persons. If you have parents they could be stigmatized. So the family has a problem, they tell you, you are consistently creating problems. They say when you left for the bush, it was a problem, now it is a problem you come back with a child without a father. We don't get any support from fathers or others. Families are rejecting us. Because of poverty women could accept sex work. It is hard to marry for an ex-combatant women with a child. Men are unlikely to accept us with a child. They say give the child to his father. But we cannot find the child's father. I wish we could join an association on HIV to get support from others. Families are rejecting us, because of poverty women could accept sex-work. With associations they can talk to others. In this way also we don't need to remember the past, bad past.

In the discussion both X and W agreed on the difficulties of life and questioned what reintegration meant for them. They saw themselves living within a community which was not their own as they could not go back to their own. Many were not welcomed by their families, as families typically considered joining the rebellion inappropriate and, as a result, think that these women brought shame on their families. The shame in this context was also linked to the children they brought back from the bush. Women found themselves in an untenable position within their families. Now they were living under the constant questioning gaze of the new community. They were young women with children and without any men to protect them. These characteristics created problems for their well-being and also framed their vulnerability. Having children without a father is an important problem. On the one hand, it marked them as a particular kind of women in the eyes of the community. On the other hand, the question of fatherhood was a troubling one. At least one of them knew which one of the men she had relations with in the bush was the father. They also knew other women who knew the father of their children but could not talk to them as they now were in a position of bureaucratic or political power. The combination of these factors made looking after their children very difficult. Some were going hungry for days to provide some food for their children. They had their own health problems, some of which were related to HIV, yet they did not have any resources to deal with these. Under these pressures, sex-work was a viable option, particularly in the urban environment in which they were living.

The way these relations have developed is underwritten by the assertion of gender governance after the conflict in a number of ways. Right at the end of the conflict, women were excluded from the DDR process and its resources by the manipulation of their positions in the armed groups. The DDR process itself unfolded within the existing gender framework that we have discussed in the earlier chapters. The policy is planned and implemented by people who have a traditional view of the role of women in their society. Therefore, the process begins by taking the role of women in society for granted. In this, women's concern about their reintegration and questions about their experiences during the conflict disappear, while at the same time the implications of those experiences become a new set of vulnerabilities for women in their post-conflict lives. While many people might have had reasons to feel supportive of the fighters in the bush, they were not happy to see their children, in particular daughters, dragged into the conflict. Furthermore, these post-conflict conditions experienced by women also highlight the nature of the gender-based violence in terms of its intra-ethnic aspects. Women were brought into the rebellion to support the combatants in the bush; in the post-conflict context they were not supported and were left alone to fend for themselves. The result of the commodification of women and their bodies during the conflict has not only created long-term implications for women after the conflict and enforced further commodification, but also created a cycle of inter-generational disempowerment, vulnerabilities, and problems for their children, particularly if these children are girls.

The difficulty for the government to engage with ex-combatants was highlighted by one high-ranking provincial administrator who was a CNDD–FDD ex-combatant:

> Reintegration activity is not easy for the government—a person comes back used, trying to make a normal living—to work hard daily but they are not intellectuals, it is hard to cope—there were lots of promises not honored, there is a misunderstanding. The follow-up is hard. They did

not use the money wisely it was often used on alcohol and prostitution. People blamed the ex-combatants for theft and other things, well they do. It is hard to put them together we need a strategy. My idea is to create mixed associations of ex-combatants and others or train them together. There is a big problem with the reintegration of women ex-combatants. They do not want to be reintegrated. They ask for money each month. Repatriates have the same problem. They want to stay with the culture, they do not want to work, if we organize a dance or other activities they do not come, few ex-combatants are at the organized communal work because of, they say, broken promises.

This identifies a distinction developed within the ex-combatants between those who were educated and ranked and those who were not. The latter group was simply expected to go back and normalize into the communities. The assumption behind this approach seems to be overly simplistic and not to accurately understand the state of affairs within communities. It also shows a tactical approach to ex-combatants by the leadership and the fact they do not consider everyone's position as important or as relevant as others in the post-conflict context.

The trajectory of one highly positioned regional bureaucrat highlights this point. Y was responsible for supervising the segment of a large social service provision for the entire province:

I joined the rebellion in 2002, leaving university where I was doing my 3rd year. I had two months training as a rebel. Then I was allowed to come back to the university to finalize my Rapport de Stage. This was part of the CNDD-FDD movement's strategy to have educated leaders who would be useful after the war. Once I came back I finished my studies. I graduated as an engineer in electromechanics. Thereafter I decided not to go back to the bush, it was already the time of cantonment-disarmament. My former commanding officer gave me a document I could show to the civil leaders of the movement in order to prove my political and military training. Then I came back home to teach in my commune. Aside from teaching I continued my political engagement. Two years later I was promoted to my present job in 2005. You know, in the movement, we had two categories of members. One group was made of armed members. The other group was consisted of people who were identified as political mobilizers. The president of the republic was part of this second group as politico-military leader. He has, as I do, a registration number in the rebel armed forces and he is also a political leader. He was demobilized in Muramvya at the same moment as some others like Nyongoma. Now I keep in contact with ex-combatants in the process of reintegration. I advise them to form an association to fight HIV/AIDS. As I am educated I used to teach different things to my former colleagues in the bush because most of them are not educated.

The situation described here highlights a number of dynamics which are important to note. Clearly the rebel groups had opportunities to facilitate better exit strategies for some from the conflict. The question is why they did not provide these for most women. The differentiation between those who were considered to be useful after the conflict and those who were only useful during the conflict also informed the way they approached reintegration. The realization of these distinctions by some ex-combatants on the basis of their reintegration experiences also meant that they felt they were left alone, without any help. As a result, people who came from poor families, or were without families, and those who were unmarried and young found it very difficult to engage with their communities.

A view from the other-side: community perspectives

There is no doubt that for ex-combatants, both men and women, it has been very hard to return to their communities and there were many complications that made large numbers leave their original communities and move elsewhere. As pointed out above this process has also created HIV risks associated with high alcohol consumption, sex work, and the psychological pressures of not having resources to maintain one's life. Owing to these circumstances many ex-combatants felt resentful towards their leaders and also towards their local community leaders for not helping them to reintegrate. It is therefore also useful to look at how communities perceived ex-combatants and their return. Contrary to the hopes and aspirations of many that ex-combatants should be considered and treated independent of their involvement in the conflict by their communities, for many in the same communities ex-combatants represented what happened in the country over a long period of time. They reminded those in the communities of their own experiences during the conflict. In a way the reintegration needs of each side were contradictory. Most people when thinking about ex-combatants immediately reflected on the conflict. For instance, in a discussion with a catholic priest Z in Ngozi, initially he did not want to talk about HIV but once asked about the ex-combatants returning he provided a view on the situation in the community which informs its perspective on ex-combatants:

> There has been a direct relation between war and HIV spread here. The family life has been shaken and destroyed at different levels. Brutally, relations have been cut between children and parents, between wife and husband. The reaction was also brutal. People are not able to integrate this into their lives. They lost the sense of life, and victims of many problems were not able to protect themselves. They were too far deep into these problems and they just seek to forget. Some were caught in drinking alcohol and influenced others. Many were falling into unprotected sex. People were accustomed to live in family, in their compounds and houses surrounded by fences and fields. Each family used to have a place where

they felt safe, and the traditional way of life, along with traditional neighborhood, created a space for safe and good behavior. Husband, wife and children lived altogether in one small room. How one could live well in that setting? People really had relational problems, with no intimacy and private space. Refugees had the worst situation. People lost everything. They had no food. Many women were pushed by this to prostitution in order to survive and earn some money. Added to this armed gangs attacked people and raped women all around.

There is a change due to the war. It is not easy to describe, it is psychological. We see now adults having more concern, even fear, about youth behavior. Youth do not talk at the same wavelength as their parents. After the war, youth are not the same as they were before. They have different reactions. They are now more spontaneous, quicker and violent, more daring. We now have, after the war, street children and street youth-not all of them are orphans. War caused and spread poverty and many problems followed this. We live in a complex situation.

This framing was a reference point in many of our interviews when people in communities were talking about the way they related to ex-combatants. It also frames people's views on the way they relate to female ex-combatants. For many, these women are seen as being in unfortunate circumstances and resorting most of the time to sex-work or transactional sex. However, not all the considerations are negative and exclusionary. This can be seen in the discussion with one health center nurse, A1, and B1, a specialist on HIV, in one of the national network's Gitega offices.

B1: Recently, we had a sensitization session for ex-combatants. They said to us that they had never had real information on HIV/AIDS before, except a quick session during their stay in the demobilization camp. Ex-combatants are highly vulnerable. In the workshops we organize we need to separate strategically our target groups as youth, soldiers and sex workers. We would deal with each group separately so that we are able to answer their questions. The work on HIV/AIDS continues now. But it must be intensified in target groups. Now the sensitization is not intense.

A1: I saw recently two ex-combatants in the commune here, one from Bugendana and the other was from Makebuko. They came to the health center among other patients. There is no specific service targeting only ex-combatants for sensitization or for treatment. They had many questions. Many of them are not sufficiently informed. I would say they are at high risk. They had a different life as soldiers and it could be hard for them to adapt to a new life. For instance they are not sure how to engage with women. They are not much informed about HIV/AIDS but they are very much interested in women. Their questions are generally were common to other's. They asked less informed questions than other people. This was telling me that they are less informed. Some ex-combatants, like some other young people, are using drugs. They are among the first group to use drugs. The second group would be sex-workers.

A1 also brought out an interesting angle for the discussion. She talked about men's language used to justify their behavior.

> When we talk about war and HIV/AIDS to people you see that health services for protection was difficult at the time. War increased HIV. For example in IDP camps one man could have sex with many women, many widows. Men used to say in Kirundi it is Gusambura ivyasanbutse—[to] Rehabilitate destroyed things [meaning that they, soldiers, were making sure that the community destroyed by the war is reproduced]. There are proverbs, especially for men to justify sex with many women using reference to traditional behavior. One is "Umwonga umwe wonza inyoni— Living in a swamp gets the bird hungry" or "Impfizi ntiyimirwa—Bull is never cornered." We try to discourage this and sensitize people against these.

In Bururi we talked to C1 who was a health specialist on prenatal care and HIV sensitization and to D1 who was a nurse specialized in HIV. They echoed the above and stated observations about ex-combatants.

C1: Ex-combatants, well they are demobilized now and are perceived to have money. They use the money to get wives or girlfriends. They are used to the habit of "just looking at the girl to see whether she is healthy" it is their way of verifying if they are ill or not.

D1: They have similar sexual habits now to others—people do not care about HIV, they say they will die at some point anyway. People have information but at the level of behavior change—there is no change. They talk openly about multiple wives, sex without condom, but still won't be tested. If HIV+, they say, I will die, so rather not know—there is a fear to know.

C1: Polygamy is big here but also in rural areas. Women suffer. People do not come for tests. If women are HIV+ they are chased away and blamed for the HIV.

These views show that professional services were trying to engage ex-combatants and that ex-combatants were not targeted by any specific government initiative and they had to be proactive in seeking help. Also important to mention here is the limited capacity of many of these professionals to react across their provinces due to both financial and human resource problems. It is also clear from the discussion that engaging ex-combatants with the HIV sensitization and testing is not very straightforward as being tested will confirm some of the worries of the community discussed earlier. They assume that they would be further stigmatized.

It is also important to look at how others, non-professionals, considered ex-combatants in their community. In a conversation with two HIV+ women in Ngozi they reflected on their own experiences of the conflict. They said that there was little about HIV information at the time and there was no time to talk. People did not want to leave their homes to avoid danger.

E1:   We know ex-combatants they are in our neighborhoods. They are back you see them in the hillside. They have good relations. My fear is that they will change after the money runs out. We don't really fear from them. They have houses, some are married with children may be they will abandon violence.

F1:   Now we don't see them as bad. They are getting on well in the community. They are like others. They had no information or sensitization on HIV/ AIDS. They need it. We think that they need more because they lost time in the bush. There was nothing, at least here there was a little bit sensitization.

E1:   There is a difference in their behavior. When you see them, the average person knows and fears HIV/AIDS. They don't fear it or think about protection. I think this is because of the war. They think that HIV virus is a simple thing—that it does not affect them—because there was no sensitization. You see the difference. They try and be direct—to use force. They used to go to sex workers, their behavior is different. The traditional shyness, they have no shame, no shyness.

F1:   They never think about condoms. They say "the gun shot did not kill me so HIV will not."

These views underline a dynamic social context where ex-combatants are part of social relations. Their behavior creates concerns for others but their behavior is also linked back to ex-combatants lives during the conflict. These reflections, considered together with others presented above, provide a clear set of constraints to the reintegration of ex-combatants and to different communities' engagement with them in a normal way. Communities are labeling them as ex-combatants and at the same time they are expected to normalize by moving beyond their past behavior. Here conditions for change are not supported by any structured or systematic policy intervention. The lack of such support and resources might be exacerbating cyclical behavior that is justified using the above-mentioned sayings about men's behavior.

The land issue was also one of the central resource problems for poor ex-combatants and for women in particular both for those who were coming back and for those who were made homeless due to the various pressures of the conflict. Owning land affords a person and her family a living, but owning and holding on to land are difficult for women who are left behind, coming back from the bush, or who are HIV+. G1 was divorced with two children and 48 at the time of the interview; H1 was married (a widow since 2004) with two children and 32 years old, and I1 was a younger mother of three and a widow. They were all HIV+. All three agreed that all widows have land issues.

H1:   I have a land problem, they wanted to take way. The youngest brother-in-law wanted to take the land, it is in court now and there is no appeal.

The court process began in the commune, I won it, it went to the provincial court, I won that too, and now it is in Bujumbura. My own family wants to take the land from me. My brother in-law tells me to go away and they will look after my children. The place was bought for us by my brother-in-law while we were married, I have the documents. He is rich and strong so he thinks that he can win.

G1: They said "she (I) should die she is already dead" my in-laws advised the children to chase me away because I am HIV+, life is very bad.

I1: I was chased away when my husband died. I was accused of being a sex-worker as I was not officially married. They took the kids but I have them now. I have no means to go to court. My husband bought land in Nyanza Lac (He was born in Buraza) and lived in Nyanza Lac before. His brother came to chase me away and others agreed with him as I was not married officially. The Bashingtahe asked me to go to the traditional court with cases of beer I finally abandoned this as I don't have money. When my children were with my brother-in-law he used to get them to herd cows. I was not happy with this.

H1: The second problem is I had nowhere to go so I fled to my parents house, when I returned, I found our house destroyed.

G1: When I was divorced from my husband I came to Rumonge. We were married in Songa. I had a small place. Then fled because of the war as my house was near to a military position and people try to chase me away. When I returned the house was burnt we built a make-shift place. The commune asks for taxes but I had no money. Children tried to go back to their father's land but uncles chased them away and they came back. But they treated one of my sons badly they beat him up while chasing them away. They were not well. My other son dropped out of the school, began taking drugs and he blames me. The other son joined the military, he was a child soldier, when he came back relations have been tough. It is hard to keep medications as I have little money.

These discussions highlight the complications created by women's marriage status and the way the absence of their husbands, for various reasons, creates a space for the exclusion of women and their children from family resources. This in turn creates a cycle of poverty for women, and these vulnerabilities in turn increase the risks to HIV. For instance, H1 was a widow and remarried to support herself. But by getting into a different marriage arrangement she also created a complication for the resource relations she had with her ex-husbands family. In G1's case the family clearly did not want to recognize her children's entitlements to their father's land. Here the poverty of the mother was a clear signal to the uncles as they knew that their nephews would not be able to pursue the case.

In another group discussion, with J1, K1, and L1, who were all female ex-combatants, the question of land was also a central issue. Here the issue was very much linked to the broader context of the conflict in Burundi and the dislocation it created over decades.

L1: I fled to Tanzania in 1972 with my parents, I was married in the camp. I came back during the war, we had land. When my husband dies I could not keep the land. I went away again because there was no peace. I rather fight than wait. I joined the rebellion and took gun. At first reintegration was hard and now it is better but the underlying problem that keep surfacing is land.

J1: We have wounds and similar problems. I was a 72 refugee too. I came back to Burundi. My brothers (other Burundians) told us that we are not Burundians. Other Burundians took all we had I was very angry, now we rent a house. But we used to have our own land and house. Take note if this is not settled the war will not really finish. Our land, house, wealth have been stolen. We see people (our neighbors) on our land this makes us angry. The reintegration package was small we see no progress. We want our kids to have a better life we did not go to school while other women went and had good jobs. We need land to live on and cultivate. The war cannot finish if there is no real justice.

K1: I too am a 72 refugee and I am renting a house here, I have nothing. We want to participate in training, support programs, there will be no future without help. We lived in Tanzania we know no one here. The one on our land will not welcome us. We put down our arms and we are trying to be live peacefully. We try to live together and offer friendly services in the neighborhood. It worked a little because we carried guns they see us differently. In the demobilization camps they told us to live together but those on our land are not helpful.

Conclusion

Overall, the success of the DDR process, when considered from the integration perspective that is leading to normalization of relations in the community, seems to be questionable. Ex-combatants found it difficult to integrate, in particular with their rural communities and remained in urban areas without much to do. This then led to tensions in urban areas. This kind of concentration of ex-combatants is also linked to the increased potential for gender violence. In addition to these problems ex-combatants accumulated large debts linked to their social space and also developed an aggressive attitude towards society. According to one expert who was involved in the reintegration process, at the end of the first round of distribution of reintegration packages in late 2007, the program [DDR] is seeing almost no impact on urban areas, especially heavily war-affected communes in the periphery of Bujumbura Town. The money distributed is not used towards building a new future within communities. People are either paying their debts accumulated since they were demobilized or spending it on alcohol, rather than using the income towards future personal development. These comments articulate an important criticism of the DDR process and its aims. Many ex-combatants argued that *the process did not really care about them.* The DDR process was seen merely as a process for authorities to discharge their perceived responsibility to the ex-combatants without much commitment to their overall well-being. In other words the DDR process neither acted as a "transformative social space" itself or led to the creation of these spaces within communities (Campbell and Cornish 2010: 1573).

Another issue here of course is the way communities felt that they were not ready to absorb ex-combatants in the way they have been demobilized, i.e. without the kind resources useful for their lives. Some of the discussions presented above also point out the scale of the general poverty created by the conflict in diverse communities. Many people had much less resources than they had before and they needed to build their homes and begin their lives once again. These issues were also complicated by the return of long-term refugees to the country. From this perspective ex-combatants were one part of the bigger problem many communities had to deal with.

This then leads to the question of how far the DDR process was successful in creating an economic basis of integration that allowed people to develop their own lives. On that score the record seems also to be negative. The size of the package was an issue. Also the distribution mechanisms were a problem. In some cases, the package was given out in different instalments in cash. It was easy to spend and also considering the debts incurred, most of it disappeared before it was put into a productive development. In some other cases agencies insisted on distributing the money as an in-kind contribution towards a small business project. Ex-combatants were asked to develop business plans and some of them were trained to do so. In these cases while some worked, others developed projects which would allow them to turn the in-kind contribution into quick cash to deal with their debts. At the end of the distribution process there was no follow-up process to see how to support these people in order to maintain what they might have developed from their packages.

Another critical issue for the success of any of these interventions was the time factor. The delay in making the packages available and waiting without resources increased ex-combatant's borrowing against future guaranteed earning expected from the package. However, it also increased their frustration, as discussed in the introduction. The time frame was also frustrating for the CNDRR and the government, as the process was stretching over a longer period than they thought, decreasing the ability to move on after dealing with the ex-combatants. In this sense the interventions based on in-kind delivery were difficult since, on the one hand, they were expected to be distributed faster, and, on the other, people needed to train. Arguably, the interests structuring the DDR created inherent structural problems that frustrated dealing with the actual problems that people were trying to deal with at the end of a long conflict.

Furthermore, the DDR process was an utter failure in dealing with the conditions and problems of women created by this conflict. Although CNDRR had a gender office in its organizational set-up, it certainly side-stepped many of the immediate gender problems associated with being a part of the conflict. The process also did not deal with the socio-economic context to create a resource base for women to develop ways of supporting themselves. Here the land issue is also critical. To expect women to develop their own economic engagements and support themselves is simply unrealistic in a context where gender governance empowers men in resource ownership and for decisions utilizing those resources. Beyond simply empowering men it actually dis-qualifies women from owning land. And, as discussed in Chapter 2, women without resources during the conflict had to find other ways to support themselves, and this created very harmful conditions for many. From the gender angle, the DDR was a process that ignored the gendered outcomes of the conflict as important for creating better communities. While at the same time it implicitly reasserted the traditional gender governance as a way of ordering social life.

Evaluated from the HIV/AIDS angle, the DDR was a failure at multiple levels. The overall process did not engage with the gender governance that was instrumentalized for sexual relations and creating HIV risks. Although there is no doubt that the provision of some sensitization and testing was important, this was done as a box-ticking exercise, as a technical intervention to comply with what is expected from a general DDR process. The process did not engage with the particularities of the conflict creating the HIV risks. It was general and constrained within the demobilization time frame. There was no attempt to develop a process with in-built follow-up procedures to engage with behavior change. This inherent problem with the operational set-up was exacerbated by the absence of women from the processes. Men and women did not have the space to have a discussion in context where they could listen to each other's experiences. Some men were engaged with HIV sensitization, many were not, though they all generally sat through HIV/AIDS sessions. From the women's perspective they were left alone to deal with their own problems. Many ended up doing sex-work or being exposed to further vio-lence within their communities, as communities were not trained or educated about the lives of these women during the conflict. In other words, the DDR process missed the community part of the reintegration. It had nothing to say about the many communities that had disintegrated because of the war and how this made women vulnerable, as discussed by many interviewees. These people were expected to adapt to the new reality. Moreover, not only did the DDR not deal with the HIV risks created during the conflict and problems associated with these risks, but it created further vulnerabilities as a result of the way it functioned. The delays in distribution of packages created social contexts where ex-combatants met women engaging in transactional sex. This undoubtedly increased HIV risks.

6 International expert knowledge and its production

The relationship between conflict and HIV/AIDS

In the preceding chapters I have considered the intersections of people's lives, conflict, and HIV/AIDS. This aimed at looking at the disjuncture between people's experiences and the international policies targeting them. Furthermore, the way this disjuncture in both the conflict and the post-conflict contexts potentially creates further risks of HIV. This chapter adds another layer to the discussion by looking at the knowledge claims both underwriting existing policy frameworks and also influencing what should be seen as the relevant knowledge in this field. This is an important discussion as the boundaries set for research is embedded in a particular kind of knowledge, and it projects what should be seen as relevant for policy frameworks. As I discussed in the introduction the relationship between conflict, sexual violence, and the spread of HIV is a serious concern for international policy makers, and the relationship between conflict and HIV has been considered an international security problem (USIP 2001; Elbe 2002, 2009; Singer 2002; Ostergard 2002; Peterson 2002; Heymann 2003; Altman 2003). However, the relationship identified between conflict and HIV/AIDS has also been questioned by many (Spiegel 2004). One particularly controversial issue has been how to assess the relationship for policy purposes given the unsettled and unpredictable conflict contexts and the fact that HIV/AIDS is still a stigmatized disease. These problems are further compounded by the difficulties faced by research conducted in conflict contexts in unpacking the nature and implications of sexual violence and its possible links to HIV. Of course, there is no doubt that good policies will rely on good information and knowledge. However, the relationship between policy making and the knowledge production supporting particular policies is not straightforward. The nature of what constitutes policy relevant knowledge continues to be hotly debated, with debates on the nature of such knowledge becoming more common in evidence-based policy (Hammersley 1995; Mullen *et al.* 2005; Kiefer *et al.* 2005; Oakley *et al.* 2005). This chapter looks at this ongoing debate by considering the kind of knowledge that can be evidential for policy making in the context of the debate on conflict and HIV/AIDS. It is also concerned with the way particular methods are seen as relevant for evidence-based policy in this context.

In a paper published in the *Lancet* entitled 'Prevalence of HIV infection in conflict-affected and displaced people in seven sub-Saharan African countries: a systemic review' Paul Spiegel and his colleagues provide an authoritative review of the existing literature on the link between conflict and HIV prevalence in Africa. In addition, both the position of the *Lancet* as one of the most important international medical journals publishing research on health and diseases and the position of the lead author as the senior HIV/AIDS expert in UNHCR—the UN Refugee Agency—lend authority to the paper (on another controversial issue and the *Lancet* see Dyer 2010). The paper's importance explains my focus on it here.

The paper's key conclusion is that the existing data are insufficient and of questionable quality for establishing the link between conflict and HIV prevalence. The authors state that "[g]eneralisations should be avoided, since they probably led to the original unsubstantiated assumptions that [we] investigated" (2007: 2194). The assumption they are investigating is stated early on as that "conflict, forced displacement and wide scale rape increase prevalence or that refugee's spread HIV infection in host countries" (2007: 2187). Their conclusion presents this important position while also calling for further research to produce robust data on conflict, displaced people, and HIV. Also of interest here is Spiegel's institutional interest to provide grounds to overcome the generalized "misconception that refugees' HIV rates are always higher than those in host countries" (2004: 335). In this way his aim is to counter a view that would create added stigmatization for refugees who are already disadvantaged by their status. Considering the mandate of UNHCR, which requires it to work with host governments to deal with refugee problems, the emergence of such stigma attached to refugees and other displaced people would create important impediments to its work.

Their findings question the policy environment that seems to base its policy interests on this "unsubstantiated" assumption, and the outcome of the review is the establishment of the lack of evidence in this field. Unpacking the review allows us to analyze how absence of evidence becomes evidence to dismiss the argument that is considered. In this way we can observe the relationship between particular methodological commitments and assumptions determining what is seen as relevant evidence.

To provide an analytical framework with which to consider the evidential claims in this work, I now briefly introduce philosopher Nancy Cartwright's work on the use of evidence. She looks at the issue from "the point of view of the evidence user" (2008). The approach is an attempt to turn the conventional evidence debates around. These debates typically focus on whether we have enough evidence for informing policy, or on what kinds of methodology produce *good-quality* evidence for policy in general (Petticrew and Roberts 2007; Seckinelgin 2007). Cartwright argues that typically evidence guidelines "tell us what counts as good science, not how to use that science to arrive at good policy" (2008: 4). In other words she is concerned with the question of how a user chooses from various kinds of knowledge to inform policy. How can users decide among facts as "[they] want … as evidence only those that are relevant to the policy" (2008: 5)? The relevance of evidence is important since we need to know that the evidence we choose will be relevant to the aims of the policy users. Here Cartwright suggests that one of the central concerns of the users is policy effectiveness: "will the proposed policy produce the targeted outcomes were it to be implemented in the targeted setting in the way it would in fact be implemented" (2008: 5). While acknowledging that there are three important issues in considering evidence for users namely "quality, relevance and evaluation" she argues that the second of these seems to be the starting point for a user (2008: 6). The question of relevance, "when does an established result bear on a policy prediction and how does it do so? (2008: 6)" is a central starting point. It considers the question of relevance as a function of the way policy makers consider what can be effective in a given policy field. This then also raises the question of quality of evidence in considering what kinds of methodology provide relevant evidence in this situation. Cartwright's position follows her previous work and focuses on causal models (2007). She argues that "when we buy a policy we are betting on a causal model, willy-nilly, whether we wish to think about it or not." In other words, causal models are present implicitly or explicitly in evidence and the policies such evidence supports. In this the policy user requires evidence that has a causal story that is relevant for the outcomes of the policy that is going to be implemented. The reason policy makers are interested in a causal story or model is because it tells the policy maker about the mechanisms that underlie the relationship they are interested in. This then facilitates their thinking about what to do about the relationship, and how to intervene in the situation.

Policy makers are not interested in general evidence but in a particular kind that will serve their interests for a particular policy and its outcomes. The research producing evidence will have to produce knowledge that can be linked to reference points that are part of the policy maker's view and needs. This perspective is particularly relevant here, since the *Lancet* review reflects concerns that are implicit in Spiegel's overall orientation and that are also evident in his earlier publications on the issue of the lack of coherent knowledge in this field (Spiegel and Nankoe 2004). Cartwright proposes a framework that can be used as a basis to evaluate the causal methods used in evidential discussion. It begins from the policy end of the process. It first considers the nature of evidence required rather than deciding on some pre-established method of evidence production. In this way her position allows one to consider the relationship between the kind of evidence that is required by different policy makers, contexts, and the implications of such demands on the way one considers quality of evidence. From the point of overall policy context I would like to push Cartwright's model a bit further. While her approach is useful in looking at the discussion from the user's position, here policy makers, there is also a need to introduce the position of those who will be targeted by a given policy. The perceptions of the target groups in relation to the evidence produced about them within parameters set to meet the policy maker's needs should also be part of the evaluation process. This move raises the question of how far the evidence constructed is about a causal model that is based on the experiences of targeted people. Cartwright's framing of the discussion in terms of causal models highlights the nature of evidence as a particular product for observing and establishing certain relationships as relevant for policy. This is a critical contribution. It makes it clear that evidence at any given time is about only one of the possible causal links that can be observed in a set of relations. In this sense there are multiple causal stories that can be observed about a given situation or event. To decide which of these will be relevant for the policy and policy outcomes is foremost a choice made on the basis of the policy maker's preferences. This still leaves the question open of how we decide between competing causal claims about policy relevance. Furthermore this question needs to be related to the way a particular causal model is presented as relevant and thus as evidence by the researchers; in this case how evidence for absence of evidence is presented. On what basis do researchers select causal stories to present as policy relevant? This also raises the question about the way all causal stories "relevant to the targeted effect" are considered before settling on one account (Cartwright 2008). This question brings the relationship between policy user's concerns and the evidence processes into focus.

Cartwright's position provides us with three ways to direct our concerns: (a) looking at the evidence debate from the policy maker's (user's) position allows us to consider how the relevance of evidence is constructed by the user relative to their policy effectiveness interests; (b) considering the possibility of multiple causal stories on an issue enables us to consider how these contesting causal stories are related to one other and why a given causal story is taken to be the most relevant; (c) Cartwright's evaluative criteria also allow us to consider how the chosen causal stories building the evidence come to designate the acceptable evidence in the field, which I will consider in the conclusion. The attempt is to consider the quality of evidence without being limited to the pre-established methodological criteria. It considers it's relevance in relation to other existing causal stories that are relevant to the relationships that a policy maker is interested in. These considerations also allow us to evaluate evidence and the policy based on given evidence from the perspective of the people targeted. It moves towards engaging with people's causal stories so that these can be considered as relevant evidence provided for decision-making processes.

In the following text I use this framing of the question of evidence to analyse the systematic review published by Spiegel and his colleagues in the *Lancet*. The following text is divided into three sections. The first section outlines the content of the review by highlighting the kind of causal story constructed. The aim is to unpack the implicit causal story underlying their considerations on the existence of evidence. The second section considers the way one can understand and evaluate the causal model that is constructed in their text. This is done by considering the assumptions informing their model. The third section unpacks the nature of the review's claim that there is insufficient evidence and looks at its implications. This section also raises questions about how the causal story they seek may limit future research in this field and what implications this framing has for the other causal stories that exist within the everyday lives of people. The conclusion evaluates the evidence that there is no evidence and concludes that this claim is unsustainable given the information provided to support it.

The systematic review

This section provides a general summary of Spiegel and his colleagues' review and unpacks the causal story that is built in the article. The research is a systematic review of the existing literature and data therein. The style of the analysis is consistent with the established conventions on evidence-based policy where systematic reviews are considered to be an important way of assessing the state of knowledge and the evidential quality of that knowledge (Brownson *et al.* 2003: 47–49; Dopson *et al.* 2005: 33). Consistent with this method Spiegel and his colleagues set out a criterion for the inclusion and exclusion of research they will include in this review. They identify the literature through database searches under key terms "'hiv,' 'AIDS,' 'conflict,' 'insurgency' and 'refugee'" (2007: 2187). The data on refugees are based on the existing UNHCR antenatal-care sentinel surveillance data. Further country and antenatal-care sentinel site surveillance data were accessed through UNAIDS and the WHO HIV global online database. Note that the data considered here are collected for the purposes of international agencies to construct a generalized view on the disease. In the case of the UNHCR data the situation is also more complicated. They rely on surveys and censuses conducted within their target communities. While this provides a general view it is difficult to understand the individual cases and the situation in particular contexts as their methods "do not allow for follow-up at the individual level. Although a census includes each individual it provides a 'snapshot' of the situation and quickly becomes outdated" (UNHCR 2010). Here it is important to highlight that prevalence refers to the proportion of people infected with HIV within a particular population at a given time and incidence is the new HIV infections that are observed in a population at a given time. While methods assess prevalence rates in particular communities in a given period, it would be harder to see how the prevalence rates change over time as the target populations assessed might be changing due to dynamics of conflicts or movement of people. Here, in order to overcome this situation, it seems the review is attempting to use prevalence data from agencies such as UNAIDS and WHO to consider the general state of prevalence in the original context of the dislocated people and compare it with the prevalence data that are created by UNHCR within its own operations. However, such comparability is a dicey process as it is not easy to establish exact origins of displaced people for which one can find coherent and in-depth prevalence data. This also complicates the assessment of incidence rates and causes of incidences. Even if the prevalence rate could be established in a refugee camp at a given period it seems that there is a challenge to assess incidence rates and their causes.

Their choice of seven countries was based on countries that had a "history of widespread conflict [and] that had original data for prevalence of HIV within the past 5 years" (2007: 2188). The countries are the Democratic Republic of Congo (DRC), Southern Sudan, Rwanda, Uganda, Sierra Leone, Somalia, and Burundi. The selection criteria found "293 articles and reports including refugee surveys 145 of these were providing data for prevalence of HIV infection and 88 had original data, out of these 65 had original data" on the seven countries chosen. This group included "27 peer-reviewed articles, 5 grey literature/reports, 33 actual surveys including 20 refugee ones mostly conducted by UNHCR and its partners" (2007: 2188). These were then scored according to the robustness of the methodology, results, and inter-pretation provided in the analysis. At this stage the researchers had already indicated the kind of causal model they are interested in for engaging with the discussion on the link between conflict and the spread of HIV. The selection criteria for the review are framed to fit the particular kind of causal model about the relationship that the policy makers are interested in. The selected studies and the level of their analyses preclude considerations of different kinds of causal models or stories. The implicitly selected mechanism is about the relationship between conflict, displacement, and its impact on HIV at a general, national, and international, level. They are focusing on a relationship that can be generalized across countries and their experiences in conflicts. Here, the model considered also reflects the position of international policy actor(s) that function across conflicts and countries.

The review moves on to look at each conflict on the basis of the selected studies. The analysis faces a common problem that the data available are not very comprehensive. Most available prevalence data either pre-date the con-flict or do not relate to the area where conflicts have been part of life for extended periods of time. According to the study, for instance in DRC "there have been no reliable data from the east, which has been affected by the conflict" (2189). While providing data on the Sudanese refugees in Kenya and Uganda, it is pointed out that "no data exist for the immediate surrounding host population" thus they look at the data from the nearest available com-munity. The data that are available on the Sudanese refugees appear to be very limited. It is pointed out that "no data exist from mostly rural areas of southern Sudan" (2190). They then look at the data from Rwanda on the conditions and point out that they are able to assess the general decline or rise in the prevalence rates based on antenatal-care sentinel data (2190). In this country context they are more concerned about data which would help them to understand the relationship between wide-scale rape during the gen-ocide and HIV prevalence. Once more it is argued that the data do not allow them to ascertain the link. On the issue of Rwandan refugees and their impact on HIV prevalence, they argue that "data for the prevalence of HIV infection in refugees are scarce" (2191). They consider the limited data available and the result again seems to be inconclusive. This pattern of questions about the availability of data and the kind of data that is available to arrive at an understanding of the relationship between conflict, displacement, and HIV prevalence is repeated in the case of Uganda and Sierra Leone. In the case of Somalia "few data were available before the 2004 countrywide antenatal-care sentinel surveillance survey ... which showed a national prevalence of HIV infection of 0.9%" with regional variations. The prevalence rates in neighboring countries are much higher "19% in Jijiga, Ethiopia (2001), 11% in Garissa, Kenya (2004)" (2191). When considering Burundi they point out that "conflict began when the country had fairly high rates of HIV infection that were higher in the capital cities than outside; prevalence was similar to that in Uganda and Rwanda" (2192). Furthermore the data seem to suggest that prevalence rates changed in Bujumbura and in the rural parts of the country in the 1990s. In terms of the state of prevalence among refugees it is argued that there are no data on them prior to 2001 and 2003. It is also pointed out that there were no available data for Burundi refugees' original communities. One reason given for this was as the semiurban location of sentinel sites (2192). However, before they begin with the discussion they also point out that the overall prevalence rates in "12 sets of refugee camps, nine (75%) had a lower prevalence of HIV infection, two (17%) a similar prevalence and one (8%) a higher prevalence than their respective communities" (2192). It is not clear whether these camps are looked at in relation to Burundi or whether they represent groups of camps looked at closely for each of the countries considered. There is a lack of references as to how these numbers are arrived at.

At this stage the causal model they are interested in becomes much clearer. The model they are concerned with is one which would demonstrate a statistical relationship between a conflict, dislocation, and the spread of HIV among those displaced or those receiving the displaced people as populations. Furthermore, these statistically established relations are considered as mechanisms in each context which are also implicitly required for comparability among conflict contexts. These mechanisms are taken to demonstrate that there is a general causal model that links conflict with HIV. The existence of such mechanisms then underwrites the causal model they would consider as evidence in this argument.

The next question we face here is the following: what do these data allow Spiegel and his colleagues to say about the argument? The research has two important overall points: (a) "there is insufficient evidence that HIV transmission increases in populations affected by conflict" and (b) there are "insufficient data to conclude that refugees fleeing conflict have a higher prevalence of HIV infection than do their surrounding communities" (2192). They then discuss the nature of data and collection during conflicts and how it becomes difficult to construct reliable evidence on these bases. Here, they recognize the possibility of the relationship between conflict and the spread of HIV as some of the cases suggest such a possibility, i.e., in Uganda, Sudan, and Sierra Leone. However, they insist that "there are no data to show that conflict increased the prevalence of HIV infection in the seven African countries studied" (2192). Again here the causal model considered is clearly linked with the possibility of comparing the relations of conflict and HIV across contexts. This argument is followed by a set of reasons that are given to explain why the link may not exist. The first focuses on the state of HIV prevalence in a number of countries at the start of the conflict; here it is argued that if the levels were low at the time they might have stayed low due to the conflict. This is in turn explained by a second reason about the actual impact of conflict: "mass killings, forced displacement, and hiding can lower the incidence of infections and consensual exposures and reduce social networks in which individuals might be exposed to HIV" (2192). It is also argued that this might be true for the refugees. This is explained by a third reason the "prevalence of HIV infection is lower in rural areas, from where most of the refugees in these countries came than in urban areas" (2192). Then the example of the eastern DRC is given as a case which diverges from this outlook. In terms of the relationship between refugees and the host communities they argue that "refugee's prevalence of HIV infection increases over time towards that of the host communities. There is no evidence that refugees exacerbate the HIV epidemic in host countries" (2192). They then use the generally observed urban–rural difference in prevalence rates and the fact that most refugees originate from rural areas to explain why, for instance, the prevalence rates might have declined in a number of countries independent of the state of conflict and the fact that refugees were coming from high prevalence countries. Here they are distinguishing prevalence rates in a country overall and the differences observed according to the original location of the refugees. They also explain at length the difficulty of linking incidents of rape with HIV infection for a number of important reasons, including problems of assessing actual numbers of rape, questions about accurate reporting due to the sensitivity of individuals, and not having information about the actual HIV status of rapists. While they consider the importance of rape they seem to be arguing that at least in the case of DRC and Sierra Leone that there is no evidence to show the link, and in fact the data demonstrate that there is no "significant difference between the prevalence in western and eastern regions [of DRC]" where the conflict is centered (2193). They also point out that there are not enough data to discuss the hypothesis that post-conflict periods might increase vulnerability for infection. And they call for further studies to be conducted. Before concluding their systematic review, Spiegel and his colleagues discuss the strengths and limitations of their work. However, there is no acknowledgment that the causal model they use to consider the hypothesis limits the discussion to the kind of mechanisms they are focusing on. In considering the available data in each conflict context they point out that the data are insufficient to provide an overall view about a mechanism that can apply in all cases. In this discussion it is not clear how they consider other available causal stories about the potential link between conflict and the spread of HIV. The interesting issue here is the fact that the review seems to consider some other causal models so long as they are relevant in their methodological constructions to the causal model considered by the review rather than considering them in terms of whether they are relevant for the postulated relationship between conflict and HIV/AIDS.

Most of the discussion here is related to the limitations of data available. In their conclusion they highlight the lack of reliable data to support the original argument, although they sympathize with the underlying reasons why such links might have been considered "to expect that incidence of HIV infection will be high in survivors of conflict and rape is understandable. However, these assumptions were not rigorously scrutinized and there were insufficient data" (2194). They caution that "[G]eneralisations should be avoided, since they probably led to the original unsubstantiated assumptions that we investigated" (2194). They also argue that there are important questions about what is known about the transmission mechanisms among people within displaced communities. The argument is effectively saying that we are unable to find data in relation to the mechanism we are assuming to underwrite a potential link between conflict and the spread of HIV in general. The implications of this argument are far reaching and I will come back to these later. Here the reader faces a central question: how does one need to understand the outcome of this systemic review? How do we evaluate its conclusions?

How do we evaluate its conclusions?

The authors dismiss the argument that there is evidence linking conflict with HIV spread. First at the beginning of their discussion and then again at the end of the article as a statement that it is not sufficiently scrutinized and is too general. It appears, however, that this dismissal is based on the limited data presented in the article. The implicit justification in the dismissal relies on a set of assumptions. These are also informing choice of favored methodologies used in the repeated surveys which are then selected to create the corpus of the reviewed studies. The dismissal is legitimated by this methodological selection. The causal story we have at the end of the article is about implicit assumptions about the mechanisms that are assumed to be relevant if the authors were to agree with the argument. Here we have assumptions about (a) the nature of epidemic in countries in conflict, (b) sexual relations between refugees and host communities, and (c) the impact of the urban–rural divide in considering characteristics/distribution of HIV prevalence and on the nature of the potential link between conflict, displacement, and HIV. These provide reference points to ascertain the possibility of the assumed relationship.

While these assumptions frame the story they also frame what the nature of the problem is. Thus the review is trying to find the mechanism that would be compatible with this framing to understand whether the relationship exists. The mechanism that is of interest to the review assumes the relationship is prevalent at a population level that can also be observed across various conflicts. Here population seems to indicate a group larger than people in particular conflicts. It pertains to people exposed to conflicts in all cases considered. In this section I will look at these assumptions that frame the causal story. This will allow us to look at the justifications for the dismissal. The section is divided into subsections relevant to focus on particular assumptions and their implications.

Nature of epidemic in conflict

In considering the link between conflict and the spread of HIV it is pointed out that this will be dependent on the state of the epidemic in a given context. Three cases are considered, Uganda in 1978–79, Guinea-Bissau from 1963 to 1974 during the independence struggle, and the war in southern Sudan, as examples where a certain link between conflict and the spread of HIV into areas unaffected before mobilization is observed (2192). But then again dismissed since there are "no data to show that conflict increased the prevalence of HIV infection in the seven African countries studied in this article" (2192). It is not clear what the grounds are for this dismissal other than a claim that there are no data in all cases reviewed. The cases considered seem to suggest to the authors that there might be a link in particular contexts. Here the argument ignores this particular angle in an attempt to provide a statement for conflicts in general.

The next argument is also rather confusing. In trying to explain the situation for DRC, south Sudan, Sierra Leone, and Somalia, the logic of the stages of the epidemic is used once more. It is argued that these countries entered conflict at the time when infection rates were low. The view on the infection rates as low seems to be an assertion. For instance, it is pointed out that "until recently there have been no reliable data from the east which has been affected by conflict" (2189). The data available for DRC showing the state of affairs in DRC relates to the western part of the country. However, considering that people displaced are from the east how do we assess whether they had high or low levels of infection? This is also what the authors admit when they point out that "there are no data from the areas of origin and asylum at the time the refugees fled from these countries" (2192). Therefore, it is not accurate to assert arguments based on low-level prevalence based on the logic of the early state of the epidemic.

Furthermore, in order to elaborate another set of reasons as to why there might not be a link, the authors provide a set of displacement-related reasons, as described earlier, and argue that due to the break-up of social networks where people are exposed, the incidence of infections might have been limited.

These assumptions are also questionable. They seem to consider, implicitly, a particular kind of consensual sex as the main concern for HIV infection in general and ignore that even displaced people can create new social networks within which sex could take place. Besides, in a conflict context the concern is not only with consensual sex but also with intensified sexual violence. These displacement-related arguments are presented as "plausible explanations" (2192) without unpacking what makes them plausible in these contexts. Who are they plausible for? Looking at the data presented for each of these countries and considering the assumptions underwriting their analysis, it is clear that what is considered is far from being plausible. Here asserting their assumptions with an overall plausibility claim, they are ignoring the existence of other possible causal stories on these issues.

Sexual behavior

Another way to consider this situation is to look at the arguments about the relationship between refugees and their host communities. Although it is stated that there are no accurate data the authors support the view that "there is no evidence that refugees exacerbate the HIV epidemic in host communities" (2192). This seems to be again an assertion. There are no data according to the authors to know what the level of HIV infection was among the refuges when they arrived and also since it is not known what the levels were in their host communities, it is hard to know what the direction of the impact is. As the four countries they focused on here are assumed to have a low level of infection, the argument suggests that over time refugee "prevalence of HIV infection increases towards that of the host communities" (2192). This only points out that refugees are clearly sexually active, contrary to what the authors have been assuming. This is not saying much about who the refugees have sex with and how. Thus it is not possible to explain the convergence of prevalence rates and causes of such an outcome. The increased rates may not have links with the host communities but be due to the movement of groups of refugees between camps or communities and their original countries as some people participate intermittently in ongoing conflicts (see Rowley *et al.* 2008). In terms of their refusal to think about whether refugees exacerbate the disease in host communities, there is a problem. On the one hand they are arguing that all these people are coming from low-infection rural areas and therefore they are unlikely to infect more. While on the other they are arguing that the host communities have higher infection rates even though most of these places are also rural communities. Here we have a problem in terms of this rural–urban divide discussion used as an analytical category as a part of the mechanism they are considering within their causal model. The accuracy of this urban–rural divide and assumed distribution of people between these spaces can be questioned, as in conflict and post-conflict contexts people are mobile and move between urban/semi-urban spaces and rural areas depending on the changing nature of conflicts.

Looking at the prevalence rates that are constructed on the basis of a priori categorical framing of urban and rural will not provide sound bases to consider the HIV outlook in many conflict contexts unless there is an accurate way of assessing the way communities mixed and dispersed in conflict and post-conflict periods.

Another problem area is the way the potential rape incidents during the Rwandan genocide are analysed. After pointing out the unreliability of the data, the review compares two large-scale reports. The one which is unpublished seems to suggest that 70 percent of 1125 female survivors were HIV+. Then they look at a later research from 1997 that surveyed 4800 women. This reports that only 2.2 percent were raped and of these 15 percent were HIV positive compared with 11 percent in women not raped. It is not clear when they compare the results of these two reports whether women who are surveyed are the same kind of group. Given that the first report is produced by AVEGA the largest genocide survivors organization created by surviving women immediately after the genocide, their report might have focused on a particular group of people while the latter report is based on a national population-based seropositivity survey which might not have been targeting the same group. Furthermore, it is difficult to get self-reporting on rape through large-scale surveys (Koss 1992; Hynes *et al.* 2004: 317–18, Rowley *et al.* 2008: 14, Steiner *et al.* 2009). Given that this was also a national enterprise it might have very well acted as a barrier for women to report their experiences, while a specialized organization focusing on the survivors might get a better sense of the situation. These concerns might be brushed aside as speculative. However, there is a general problem with the way this issue is approached in the review. The implication of the analysis seems to be that conflict-induced rape was not more common or impacted women's lives more in terms of HIV than the general state of HIV prevalence. Although they emphasize the abhorrence of rape, they seem to consider this issue so long as it matters for the HIV discussion. How do we decide when rape matters for policy concerns? How can one decide what is the acceptable rate of rape for it to be considered as an issue for women that needs to be tackled. Does rape in this context have to be linked with high levels of HIV infection at the population level to be considered significant? (Jewkes 2007). Here the choice of not to concentrate on these numbers is a part of the causal model that has been framing the review. These numbers do not show a significant change, thus from the position of a population they do not contribute to the discussion. However, these numbers signify experiences that are about conflict, rape, and HIV. They represent divergent causal stories to the one that is considered at the population level. Again the review engages with only some "relevant" causes.

Urban–rural divide

In looking at the limitations of the research, the researchers caution against strong assertions related to the estimates of levels of infection in countries.

Here there are two central reasons for the caution. One, they point out that "there is a limited time-trend data" in most of the countries studied (2193). As a result, it is argued that there is an ambiguity in understanding the level of infections at the beginning of various conflicts and the reduction (or increase) during the conflict. In addition this lack of data makes it hard to establish the changing relationship in terms of HIV infections between host communities and refugees. The second reason is linked to the methods of assessment. They point out that in addition to various biases based on age, geographical considerations, and the urban–rural divide, the different outcomes observed in the measurements are based on ante-natal clinics and general population surveys. They argue that the former sites tend to produce higher rates than the latter. These limitations suggest that "comparisons [among countries] should be made cautiously" (2193). Independent of this caution and the recognized limitations of available data and the methods used in gathering it, the research relies on comparisons and generalizations. In dismissing the argument the review asserts that given the low levels of infection in rural areas "it is unlikely that the relationship between refugees and local populations increase HIV infections" (2193). Here the reader has a dilemma, either there is strong general evidence to assert this, independent of the lack of data, in individual countries or this is a spurious claim on the basis of the recognized limitations of the research. Another problem in relation to the comparison is the assumption implicit in looking at Rwanda and then linking the Rwandese infection pattern to Burundi to suggest that this might be a regional pattern (2193). It is not clear on what basis this comparison is produced. It seems that in conducting the systematic review the authors are implicitly assuming a uniform pattern of sexual relations across the countries analysed. This is clearly a problem given that the countries analysed have different socio-cultural and economic structures influencing gender relations that regulate sexual relations. Furthermore, considering the characteristics of the conflicts in each country, these countries are unlikely to have similar infection patterns.

The assumptions considered here on the nature of conflicts, sexual behavior, urban–rural divide influencing characteristics/distribution of HIV prevalence and on the nature of the potential link between conflict, displacement, and HIV both set the reference points and content of the assumed relationship. This construction and the measurement of the relations through those reference points then inform the mechanisms that are considered as a causal story that might have been supported by the data. The systematic review is guided by these categorical assumptions that are aimed at looking at a generalizable story. It is this view, that if there is a link it should be observable in all conflict contexts according to a similar register that is implicitly tested. There are a number of important issues here: (a) while the data across seven conflict contexts are considered according to their methodologies to see whether the review's causal story is confirmed, clearly the original purpose of the data collection and research in these different works would have been to provide a different kind of causal story from the one which is attempted in this systematic review; (b) while the methodological selection creates grounds for comparability of the data, it appears that the contextual details of the research might jeopardize comparability across different conflicts; (c) the framing assumptions are focusing on comparability across conflicts to see whether the relationship can be considered or not; to do this the potential validity of the review's assumptions in a given context are ignored; (d) these constraints related to the methodological selection criteria and the assumptions framing the overall research ignore any other causal story that might inform the validity discussion outside the assumptions of the review. Considering the relationship between evidence and user provided by Cartwright, here assumptions are revealing preferences for a particular kind of user/policy maker. The mechanisms that are considered in the causal model are about the possibility of generalized interventions by international actors. Therefore, the evidence sought needs to support this kind of interest.

In order to take the discussion a step further one of the central questions is in what ways the nature of the data considered provide evidential justifications in the context of a conflict–HIV relationship as highlighted in the review? This is linked to the more general question of what is meant by evidence in this review. Once these are considered the conclusion statement that there is no evidence should be reconsidered.

The nature of evidence

The research in its main conclusion argues that we are unable to falsify the null hypothesis that there is no link between conflict and HIV/AIDS. This then leads to the argument that there is insufficient evidence for the evidential discussion to take place about the argument. As a result we cannot consider the argument whether there is a link. Thus it is argued that there is a need for further research to produce evidence to test the hypothesis. Here it is important to understand: what this claim produces This conclusion that there is insufficient evidence to engage in the discussion needs to be scrutinized. It is true that there are insufficient data in the particular format this review is considering. It does not immediately mean that there is no evidence in general. It might suggest that the way the evidence framework is constructed in this particular review is not the appropriate framing for producing evidence in this area. Therefore, it is important to unpack what kind of evidence the available data produce and what is meant by evidence in the context of this review.

The idea of evidence that is relevant for the research is implicit in the way the researchers constructed their selection criteria for inclusion and exclusion of a particular kind of study. In their research, they used a number of key words to trace studies. These key words included HIV, AIDS, war insurgency, conflict, and refugees (2187). Once the studies were put together they carried out further selection, choosing works with data on the prevalence of HIV infections. The next step from this group was to select those studies that provided original data on HIV prevalence. Here the verification of original data is linked to the data produced on the basis of survey methods: either antenatal-care sentinel surveillance or general population-based studies. Then the data are carefully considered by two epidemiologists in the team looking at "sample size and power, sampling method, testing algorithm, results and interpretation of the data" and then papers were ranked for further selection (2188). This further focusing based on looking at the way "the sampling method or testing algorithm" was consistent with "the guidelines" (2189). It is clear that the review is interested in a population-wide view on the prevalence of HIV infection. In this context this means that the study is interested in data that can show the relationship between conflict and HIV at a population level. In this they were also considering how far, if such a relationship exists within the data, it can be generalizable. In order to secure this they look at population-based research and focus on research that used large-scale survey methods. The generalizability is at two levels, whether conflict impacts the prevalence of HIV in a general population or not. Then, the consideration is about whether this relationship can be observed across different conflicts in Africa. This brings in their country selection criteria to include countries "with widespread conflict" and "those countries where there is original data for prevalence of HIV infection within the past 5 years" (2188). Again here their concern about the potential generalizability of the existence of a relationship between conflict and HIV, or not, seems to be the driving focus. In other words, for them if there is evidence for the relationship then it should demonstrate the relationship at a population level and across conflicts. Here the possibility of an assumed link is tested in particular terms that ignore country-specific characteristics of violence and conflict. This also frames the nature of evidence the review produces. The nature of the relationship which is considered seems to assume, as discussed in the previous section, that there are a limited number of pathways for conflict and HIV to be linked. It is at these limited points around conflict-based violence, rape, and the impact of refugees on host populations that diverse conflicts are compared as a group. However, even if these limited reference points are accepted, each conflict will have a different way of creating these conditions. In other words, it is not clear how such a diverse conflict context can be analysed as a group to test this hypothesis at a general level.

Furthermore, by requiring the availability of data on HIV prevalence within the last five years for conflicts to be included in the review, the study appears to use this as a ground for comparability. Here the relationship between conflict and HIV is assessed on the basis of whether there has been any change in HIV infection rates in the last five years in the conflict countries. There are two issues here. One, the review points out that there are very little base line data on HIV infections within many communities at the beginning of a number of these conflicts. Thus, the data about the last five years will provide a speculative comparison for the assessment at best. Two, the conflicts are historically disparate and follow different timelines. For instance, it is pointed out that there was political instability in "Rwanda from 1990 to 2002, with genocide in 1994. Uganda underwent conflict in 1978–79 ... and the present conflict in Uganda that began in 1988. The civil war in Sierra Leone between 1991 and 2002 ... In Somalia, the civil war officially lasted from 1989 to 2002. Burundi has had a low-intensity conflict with intermittent high-intensity episodes since 1991" (2188). It seems that these qualitatively different conflicts are compared with each other under assumptions about the way conflicts are supposed to be linked with HIV in general. However, the impact of the timeline given for instance for Rwanda, and the implications of genocide are different from what is described as the conflict situation in Burundi. Independent of these differences the review considers these cases comparatively (2192). The review argues that in "Burundi ... prevalence was similar to that in Uganda and Rwanda" when conflict began (2192). This is rather confusing was it similar to Uganda and Rwanda at the beginning of their conflict? Or was it similar to these countries at the time Burundian conflict began around 1991 on the timeline used by the review? If it is the former the existence of accurate data about the Ugandan conflict in 1978 and in the early 1980s on HIV is dismissed by the review itself (2191). Then it is not clear whether the comparison with Rwanda is in relation to 1991 as a base or to 1994 to the genocide. Considering the nature and particularities of the Ugandan conflict, if the comparison with Burundi is taking 1991 as the base line is the comparison with Uganda overall or does it only include the areas where the conflict has been focused? The review considers the available data on Uganda by comparing the change in prevalence across Uganda. It is pointed out that "the prevalence of infection in northern Uganda, as in the rest of the country, fell during the 1990s and early 2000s" (2191). They also suggest that the prevalence might be rising now. If the rates were falling in the 1990s according to the assessments, does this fall report the situation during the conflict after 1988? Furthermore, they point out that although "the intensity of conflict increased from 1996 onwards, trends from 1998 to 2003 showed a larger decrease in Gulu" (2191). Could this be related to the characteristics of the conflict in Northern Uganda, or even how far people had access to health services where some of the surveys producing this data were conducted? The review still maintains that "prevalence remains high in northern Uganda in 2002, Gulu had the highest prevalence of all sentinel sites in Uganda" (2191). If this is the case, there needs to be an explanation as to why Gulu has this prevalence profile, how it is linked with the conflict, and the particular pattern of mobility of armed groups, their deployment, and the people who are destabilized in the area. The statistical mapping of prevalence rates does not seem to highlight why such prevalence rates are maintained despite earlier claims that northern Uganda demonstrated a fall in prevalence similar to the rest of the country.

The review, in producing its evidence, is not concerned with the characteristics of particular conflicts. The duration of a conflict together with its particular characteristic of troop deployments, the way they create various kinds of displacement and mobility within countries, the characteristics of people who are displaced, and the way gender relations become put under pressure in these societies influences the way a conflict might impact HIV. Also, the way conflicts end and resources are made available to the populations have an impact on the prevalence of HIV infections. These considerations have important implications for the attempted assessment of the state of the evidence but, they also present locations of mechanisms that might have a role in producing the relationship between conflict and HIV. The review does not look at these complicated relationships. It takes the state of HIV infections in the available data and infers the analysis from the way the prevalence of HIV infections has changed. For instance, the way Uganda data are compared to neighboring countries demonstrates this logic (2191). Here conflict contexts are implicitly reduced to the trends observed at sentinel sites which demonstrate whether prevalence has increased or not in this logic. This is then used to infer whether conflict is a component in this change. The way the data are considered makes it hard to understand whether these cases are used as illustrative examples to highlight through which paths there is a possibility of a relationship. Or, the cases represent a coherent picture about the conflicts that can be a part of the statistical analysis. This then considers the possible relationships at the general level of the review. Leading to the dismissal of the link as there is no discernible change (or enough data to show) in the prevalence of HIV infections in most of these cases.

As it is stated in the first paragraph of the review, the aim of the review is to question "the common belief that conflict fuels HIV/AIDS epidemic and consequently refugees and internally displaced placed people fleeing humanitarian emergencies have a high prevalence of HIV infection" (2187). In order to do this the review goes through various studies and demonstrates that data are not statistically significant, at the conventional 95 percent level, and fails to falsify what appears to be their null hypothesis that there is no link between conflict, displacement and the spread of HIV. As the observed data could not demonstrate that the assumed link does not exist, the review argues that there is insufficient evidence. There are a number of outcomes: the failure to reject the null hypothesis does not really help their conclusions. The absence of evidence considered in this manner does not necessarily lead to the conclusion of the dismissal of the argument. Insufficient evidence to falsify does not mean that there is no evidence. It means that we don't know. The logical step here should have asked whether this is the best way to consider the hypothesis. Clearly the nature of evidence that seems to be insufficient is linked with the generalizable causal mechanisms assumed in the causal model they are interested in. However, this does not mean that there are no other causal stories highlighting mechanisms that might be more relevant for considering the link between conflict, displacement, and the spread of HIV. In particular, considering that some of the studies that are deemed to be statistically insignificant with levels lower than 95 percent seems to suggest some (weaker) support for the claim that there is a link between conflict and HIV/ AIDS. Particularly if these lower cases are considered within sub-populations rather than in relation to the significance levels relevant for overall population.

Some of these should have led the researchers to reconsider the relevance of the selection criteria for inclusion and exclusion used and the assumptions leading the review. As I suggested at the end of the first section, this situation has important implications. The most important is about the burden of proof. By arguing that there is insufficient evidence to falsify, the systematic review creates a burden of proof on those who think that there is a link. In order to be able to engage with the argument they have to falsify the null hypothesis, which is a stringent requirement. In particular, what they called insufficient data includes data which would help to show the link. Furthermore, the systematic review focuses the possibility of dealing with the burden of proof on a particular kind of knowledge in a given format. The assumptions framing Spiegel and his colleague's interests in particular mechanisms, thus establishing a set causal model, become the grounds for considering the relevance of future research and evidence on this issue.

Conclusion

I have argued here that it is important to evaluate the evidence that there is no evidence. Contesting the existence of evidence to consider whether there is a relationship between conflict and HIV, even before one can discuss the nature of the relationship, creates an understanding of the situation as if no knowledge exists on the issue. This might suggest that policy in this area needs to build the knowledge base, but in the mean time to address people's needs policy will be articulated within a certain vacuum. Considering the systematic review through the use of evidence framing provided by Nancy Cartwright, this view of evidence leading the review becomes unsafe and inaccurate. By way of conclusion, I will provide reasons for this evaluation.

If we go back to the three points in the introduction that are derived from Cartwright's theoretical framework, we can consider the limitations of the evidence that the review produced. This will also suggest that the evidence is far from being a generalizable statement about the relationship that exists or not between conflict and HIV/AIDS. The first contribution we derived from Cartwright's position was to consider evidence in relation to some user policy maker rather than it being an independent product. In unpacking the review, we demonstrated that the causal story, which is considered to assess whether a mechanism between conflict and HIV/AIDS exists, suggests that the review was interested in the potential relationship from a position of international policy making. If we pose the question Cartwright has "when does an established result bear on a policy prediction and how does it do so?", we have the starting point for the causal model that was of interest to Spiegel and his colleagues. Here, Spiegel's institutional interest is to provide grounds to overcome the generalized "misconception that refugees' HIV rates are always higher than those in host countries" (2004: 335). In this way his aim is to counter this debate that would create added stigmatization for refugees who are already disadvantaged by their status. Thus, the relevance of evidence considered has focused the debate in such a way that the cases considered had to demonstrate significant relations that can be applied across all the cases in a comparative manner. Therefore, the evidence that they were interested in seems to be only on those things which will make sense as evidence for policy makers at the international level. This leaves all other policy concerns such as sexual violence and the evidence related to people's experiences and observations presenting different mechanisms and causal stories outside the review.

Considered from the position of the evidence produced and its relationship with other causal stories in this area relevant to the argument, the review seems to have failed. The review focused on the possibility of observing one kind of mechanism that they were interested in. By doing so, it methodologically precluded considering other possible causal stories from consideration. This particular situation challenges the conclusion that there is an absence of evidence. It is not possible to argue for such absence if the review has not considered all relevant causal stories which might be interrelated with the relationship considered. It seems the evidence that there is an absence is accurate only from a very narrow view constructed in the review. From the broader perspective it is not clear whether such a view on absence can be sustained. On balance, the generalized claim is not evidence based as its knowledge base is limited to a narrow area. Here the failure is related to understanding the dynamic context within which multiple mechanisms at various levels create the conditions for the relationship between conflict and HIV/AIDS.

By ignoring this limitation of the evidence they have produced in the review and then concluding about the absence of evidence in general, not only do they ignore their own advice on avoiding generalizations (2007: 2194), but they create an important problem for the general policy environment. Their evidence becomes an implicit part of the policy-making process through which other causal stories are also ignored. And, as I suggested in the introduction, this is another area to consider in relation to the evidence and policies that might stem from this evidence. The net outcome in this case could be that targeted resources needed by many people in relation to conflicts and HIV/AIDS do not materialize. Tim Hope (2009) considers this as an important requirement. Following Nobel Laureate James Heckman, he argues that "before we make statements about policy selection, it is [therefore] a primary requirement that we attend to the selectivity inherent in our method of collecting data about the policy selection in question" (Hope 2009).

The analysis of this review provides a cautionary tale on evidence, its production, and the status it gains once it has been produced as a way of influencing policy processes. Here the evidence debate can be considered in line with Carol L. Bacchi's work in which she considers the way policy problems are representations of particular positions rather than being objective facts out there in the world. It is argued that representations also establish what is relevant for consideration in policy terms (Bacchi 1999, 2009). I argue that discussions on the nature of evidence required for policy within international development at present act in the same manner. They provide discussions on required evidence that represent the problem in a particular way and limit the required "type of knowledge about a topic" (Hall 1992: 291). At the end, evidence might be relevant for a particular policy actor but its relevance for those targeted by the policy could and should be questioned.

I have provided a close analysis of the way the evidence debate is constructed by paying particular attention to the link between methodologies and how they inform, once deployed, knowledge claims which then become a state of the knowledge for policy considerations. The argument points out that in order to consider validity of evidence, technical methodology considerations are one among many considerations to which policy makers needs to pay attention. The discussion highlights that (a) there is more than one kind of knowledge that can be considered for thinking about problems; (b) the relationship between policy relevance of knowledge and its relevance to people's lives needs to be considered; and (c) it raises a central question for international policy actors: given that conflict contexts differ, can there be a general evidence that underwrites the relationship between conflict and HIV/AIDS?

7 People's voices
Questions of evidence and HIV/AIDS

The research reported in the earlier chapters reveals people's perceptions and their understanding of conflict, HIV/AIDS, and the ways these interact through complex mechanisms. These experiences, when read in relation to the last chapter, raise questions about the underlying knowledge claims in the study analysed in that chapter. At its most general the question that follows is about how far the claim of absence of evidence established by Speigel *et al.* (2007) and discussed in Chapter 6 can be sustained. Their study looks at the existence of evidence for a particular hypothesis in a particular way and on that basis the claim of absence could be sustained. But, there are a number questions this raises: What counts as evidence? Or, what is the relevant evidence in this case? Furthermore this then raises the question of what is the relevant hypothesis.? The last question is about the way hypothesis is relevant or based on people's experiences of HIV and conflict. Speigel *et al.*'s work makes one think whether people's experiences are relevant for evidential discussion at all? If people's experiences are not considered as relevant for an evidential discussion on HIV/AIDS, what are the grounds on which to understand the relationship between conflict and HIV/AIDS? These concerns raise much deeper questions about the grounds of the knowledge claims that frame research into the conflict and HIV/AIDS, and about the methods that allow this knowledge to be produced.

In the last chapter I discussed the main methodological problems in the way the Speigel *et al.* study is conducted. In this chapter I ask how is it possible to ignore the existing knowledge that is within people's everyday lives. It is an important question within the overall framework of the book. As I discussed in the introduction, the research material based on the security framework raised important questions. The security framework is functioning as another top-down form of determining the limits of knowledge claims in relation to HIV/AIDS. This chapter raises epistemological questions unpacking the problems associated with this top-down framing that marginalize and exclude people's experiences/their knowledge from the discussions of evidence. In the previous chapter, another important issue was the way international actors were influencing the nature of evidence considered in this area. Here I discuss a related issue that, in addition to this filtering, there is also a methodological filtering which allows people's experiences to disappear in the discussions of HIV/AIDS.

The chapter is divided into three main sections. The first section deals with some theoretical issues on evidence, that is the way a particular kind of knowledge for use is produced. Following that, in the second section I look more closely at the way the study, a systematic review, constructs the Burundian experience and evaluates the implications of conflict for HIV/AIDS. The third section then considers Burundi from the way people talk about their experiences, and then we have the conclusion.

Evidence in context

In the previous chapter the discussion focused on the question of what kind of evidence is required to consider the relationship between conflict and HIV/AIDS. The analysis there highlights some epistemological limits to the way HIV/AIDS is approached from the international policy perspective. There are two interlinked limits here. The first is the methodological boundaries of the approach, that is, selection of research according to methods used in them, and thus limiting the way evidence can be constructed. The second limit relates to the assumptions informing the substantive components of the approach. In this, a set of social relations is prioritized to assess the relationship between conflict and HIV/AIDS. I now discuss the first limit.

The analysis in the previous chapter highlighted that the model used in the systematic review was based on a number of assumptions about what matters if we are to observe a relationship between conflict and HIV, and then looking at whether we can observe such relations at certain significant levels. Implicitly this process assumes a causal model to be verified on the basis of statistically significant results. Following this approach Spiegel *et al.*'s review concludes that they are unable to observe any significant relationship in their observations of the mechanisms and, thus, that there is no evidence on the nature of the relationship between conflict and HIV/AIDS in seven countries studied in Africa. While they ask for further research to be conducted to create data, they seem to ignore the evidence that might be available but which is not accessible to the method they prioritize in creating their model of assessment. This situation of demanding more research while ignoring a particular kind of data highlights a strong methodological commitment. The causal model they consider as relevant to the possible relations they seek to identify relies on inferential methods where certain associations between behavior and outcome need to be observed. Observation of a strong correlation in these associations suggests that there is a probable relationship to which policy makers need to pay attention in their approach to conflicts.

This approach creates the limits which are interlinked. The review method is an attempt to filter information according to the methods of research considered to be rigorous, i.e., research that is mostly based on large surveys to create the data for consideration. This creates a particular selection criterion for Spiegel *et al.*'s work. The way the collected research data are analysed creates methodological limit. It analyses what can be inferred from the data on the basis of a limited number of proxies to assess the relationships. Here the systematic review considers the relationship between conflict and HIV spread using the data they have selected. The result is neither negative nor positive. The review argues that there is not enough data to consider the hypothesis. This is divergent from many similar processes where evidence either supports the hypothesis or refutes it.

Helen E. Longino argues that:

> different aspects of one state of affairs can be taken as evidence for the same hypothesis in light of different background beliefs, and they can serve as evidence for different and even conflicting hypotheses given appropriately conflicting background beliefs.
>
> (Longino 1990: 43)

Longino's "background beliefs" are what I have here called assumptions that inform the kind of links that are seen as important for the HIV and conflict relationship. These assumptions are very much informed, as I argued in the last chapter, by international policy interests. These assumptions, background beliefs, are not just attitudes and perceptions. Longino adds that:

> background belief is an enabling condition of the reasoning process in much the same way that environmental and other conditions enable the occurrence of casual interactions ... Background beliefs function as they do because they are beliefs or assumptions about connections (actual or presumed, correlated or casual) between particular kinds of states of affairs and other kinds (of states of affairs).
>
> (Longino 1990: 44)

In short, these background beliefs affirm certain kinds of relations while ignoring others. The evidential debate, as a result, always focuses on a particular subset of the all possible relations between various states of affairs. It, therefore, follows that there should be discussion about which of the relationship(s) prioritized in any given evidence is the most relevant in a given field at a given time and for a given purpose. This then raises the question of who should evidence be relevant to? And what is the position of those targeted by these policies in relation to the framing of the relevant evidence?

As discussed in the last chapter, Nancy Cartwright's position on users of evidence elaborates on this point by bringing policy makers into sharp focus. However, it does not go so far as to consider target groups or those impacted by the policy. There are at least two reasons to require evidence to be informed by people's experiences: (a) those who are targeted have a unique epistemic view point in relation to their experiences of the problem; (b) in a given policy context ultimately those targeted have greater interest in the actual outcomes of the policies as these directly impact their lives. There is no reason to assume that the interests of the policy makers will necessarily over-lap with the interests of those who are targeted. Therefore, it is reasonable to consider difference of interests and the way these differences are based on different assumptions, background beliefs, that inform the kind of evidence that is considered to be relevant.

The background beliefs of policy actors and their views on what matters inform the kind of evidence these actors want to produce. For example, the outcomes expected from the systematic review conducted by Spiegel *et al.* provide the general base line considering whether there is a link between HIV and conflict. However, even if they were able to produce evidence to show a link, this would not have produced results to understand the contextual, everyday, relationship between conflict and HIV/AIDS. For instance, the use of social relations such as rural–urban divide and their link to HIV/AIDS create the reference points to filter what informs the knowledge on conflict and HIV/AIDS. The research then considers the intensity of the relationship between urban–rural dislocation and the intensity of HIV spread to consider the link between conflict and HIV/AIDS. The natural question that comes to mind here is how one decides which relations matter. In their analysis, the model they have has already determined for them the relations that mattered in this area. But it says nothing about how these relations were created and, for instance, about how different actors participate in these processes. The relationship between conflict and HIV/AIDS is being framed as a security problem in relation to the peacekeepers working under the UN mandate and to military and/or to other armed groups. The evidence that is demanded here does not directly relate to the country contexts or the way people experience conflicts and HIV/AIDS. The evidence is not framed to address people's questions and needs. These are not assumed to be relevant for understanding the link between conflict and HIV/AIDS.

Longino's view on background beliefs allows one to raise the question of whether the strong methodological orientation of the review and the assumptions that inform the hypothesis it considers limited discussion in such a way that the absence of discussion in the Spiegel *et al.* review becomes a one-sided discussion at best. Furthermore, there are questions about the background beliefs that lie behind choosing a particular method to construct the systematic review. For example, as the review was attempting to look at the question across seven countries it focused on data that were comparable across these countries. But it is not clear why this methodology then allows the conflict–HIV/AIDS relationship to be considered as generalized. Would this criterion for the admissibility of data be relevant if we are to consider the conflict–HIV/AIDS link outside the international policy concerns? Longino argues that "if some state of affairs is evidence for a hypothesis only in light of some further background belief or assumption, then changes in back-ground belief will result in changes in evidential status" (1990: 53). The data that are available according to Spiegel and his colleagues is partial at best and inconsistent within an individual country, let alone having cross-country coherence. The question here is about the relevance of Spiegel *et al.*'s background beliefs informing their model and the lack of justification for these background beliefs. As a result of these they are contentious. Their view on the availability of data will be different if the background beliefs on the kind of relations that are important change.

The assumptions framing the methodology of the review are a function of the background beliefs that already framed the security and HIV/AIDS discussion. They are not explanatory in relation to the experiences of people in conflict on HIV/AIDS. Arguably when Spiegel *et al.* talk about the absence of data when considering the evidence, this absence is related to the background theory that they appeal to, on security and HIV/AIDS, which developed since the late 1990s. The method is already committed to a particular position due to the assumptions underwriting their review process. As a result, this shields the discussion from questions of whether the evidence, or in the present case, the claimed absence of evidence, are the relevant ways to consider the relationship between conflict and HIV/AIDS. This is also about a model of acquiring knowledge where expert beliefs are prioritized through methodological claims. The approach is modeled to exclude knowledge based on people's everyday experiences. This model here seems to function along the lines of what Loraine Daston and Peter Galison considered to be a "mechanical objectivity" device "to eliminate the distortions introduced by this or that subjective observer" (2007: 258).

There is no doubt that in the methodology used for the systematic review, the attempt was to produce results by relying on internal validity and quantifiable cross-country analysis, both of which have a persuasive power within policy circles. However, the results will not be able to say much about the processes that might facilitate or create the various relations between conflict and HIV/AIDS. The method can only map parameters that are presumed to matter and not those underlying contextual relations establishing the mechanisms that might matter most. For instance, there is the absence of knowledge on gender and sexual relations, on the way gender norms regulate social behavior or the impacts of conflict, and how these put stress on these relations to produce particular kinds of reactions. In many contexts neither uniformed services nor women represent a homogeneous population. But by considering the military and armed group contexts as the most relevant for analysing risk in relation to HIV/AIDS, the debate ignores the everyday vulnerabilities that exist in society and how these are experienced differently by people. Clearly soldiers and armed groups are embedded in larger social contexts where their sexual behavior is formed according to various social roles they play in addition to being soldiers. There is no doubt that the military environment creates a particular masculine outlook with its own way of influencing soldiers' behavior (Enloe 2000, 2007; Elshtain 1987). A soldier, or a rebel, is also a man who is a part of a community, a family, and has other social relations. By focusing on a soldier's role de-contextualized from wider society, Speigel *et al.*'s approach ignores the way gender roles regulate people's sexual behavior. This situation is further complicated when uniformed groups are not part of the regular army but represent more diffused structures linked to various communities across a country. This is a further important limitation to the security and HIV/AIDS debates. Through its focus on the military, the security debate implicitly considers the risks to the general population as a secondary issue. The security and HIV/AIDS framework is not only unable to conceptualize the situation for those who were insecure because of their gender positions during the conflict, but it also ignores those who leave the military.

This also raises yet another question about the methodology. Since all these mechanisms will have different characteristics across countries and even within one country depending on socio-cultural groups and their intra- and inter-ethnic relations in that country, there needs to be justification as to why one needs to consider data across seven countries to assess the state of evidence. Ultimately, it seems that the reason is that the systematic review exercise is about looking for the effects of relations international experts think are relevant. It does not consider whether there are important processes linking conflict with HIV/AIDS and what might be the mechanisms of these processes. Of course it might happen that some of these relations might be related to the experts' views, but this cannot be sufficient grounds to limit what one needs to know, or to accept or to dismiss the hypothesis as important as whether conflict impacts on HIV/AIDS.

There is also another problem. It is the existence of the kind of data that should have provided a broader picture. The relevance of evidence from people and its clear link to their policy needs provides a different kind of evidence that is more contextually focused rather than analytically decontexualized. This approach gives some access to what we do not obtain from the probabilistic story that is given on the basis of measurement of statistical significance of particular relations. The alternative here is to look at what people's experiences highlight about the process and mechanisms influencing their behavior in relation to conflict and HIV/AIDS. In this, structural relations can be observed on how certain kinds of behavior are produced, how they are changed, and on the direction of change in a society, and on how conflicts stress these relations to produce change. Here the nature of evidence produced is different from the one produced by probabilistic considerations. It will be more contextual and look at pathways through which socio-cultural processes produce impact. It does not start from a comparability constraint but instead looks at the context and then considers which part of the discussion might also have been relevant in different contexts.

In the next section I shed more light on this by looking at the way Spiegel *et al.*'s systematic review to construct the Burundian case according to a particular understanding of the conflict and HIV/AIDS. This then allows us to have a clear differentiation between what is reported in this book as people's experiences of conflict and HIV/AIDS and the way international expertise is framing the discussion. To do this, I focus on one of the statements in the review that considers the nature of the conflict in Burundi and the implications of this characterization of conflict for the HIV/AIDS-related outcomes. I also focus the discussion on the material produced in relation to my research in Burundi and the interview material that reveals people's perceptions on conflict and HIV to flush out the important contrasts between the two approaches.

Burundi light: Burundi from the perspective of the Spiegel *et al.*'s review

The Spiegel *et al.* review first mentions Burundi in the description of country selection. There it is stated that "Burundi has had low-intensity conflict with intermittent high-intensity episodes since 1991" (Spiegel *et al.* 2007: 2188). It then appears a second time in the Results section. There they start the analysis of Burundi by stating that "in Burundi, conflict began when the country had fairly high rates of HIV infection that were higher in the capital cities [sic]" (2007: 2191). They argue that in time the prevalence rates in the capital, Bujumbura, declined and the rural prevalence rates "lagged behind"(2007: 2192). They then report the results of the "2003 national antenatal-care survey" showing "overall prevalence of 3.9% with 6.2% and 2.1% in urban and rural areas respectively" (2007: 2192). The results also point out that there is a problem finding data about the rural populations in Burundi. Burundi then appears for the last time in the review's discussion section. In comparing the characteristics of prevalence in Uganda, Rwanda, and Burundi at the beginning of the conflict the review tries to explain why they observed a gradual decline in prevalence in these countries over time. For comparison they use a pattern they observed in Uganda mostly in relation to areas unaffected by the conflict. The explanation they entertain focuses on the differences between urban and rural prevalence levels before people fled from their countries. The implication is that even if they were leaving a high-prevalence country like Burundi, because they were mostly from rural areas they had low-prevalence rates. Thus, the prevalence rates would have been similar to their host communities. After considering other cases and a number of issues such as sexual violence and rape used as a weapon of war in a number of countries such as DRC, Rwanda, and Sierra Leone they point out the inconclusive nature of the data on these issues. Towards the end of the discussion the review highlights constraints in collecting and analysing what seems to be limited data. Constraints include the lack of comparable "data on HIV status among refugees and their immediate surrounding communities" and also the lack of reliable time-trend data for the prevalence of HIV infection in number of countries (2007: 2193).

With these and other constraints in mind the review concludes that there is not enough evidence to understand these dynamics at present. Furthermore, it is pointed out that "to expect that incidence of HIV infection will be high in survivors of conflict and rape is understandable" (2007: 2194), but there is insufficient data to study these relations. The review frames the debate clearly in a particular manner, as discussed in the previous chapter. Here I want to focus on its approach to Burundi. The review considers the characteristics of Burundian conflict in a particular manner, and constructs the way the Burundian conflict is expected to have impacted diverse communities in the country. This is also done in a comparative manner to the other conflicts from other countries. From the way they unpack the HIV prevalence in countries, it is clear that Uganda, Rwanda, and Burundi are seen as comparable cases in terms of their HIV outlooks and in the way the conflicts might have impacted this outlook. Furthermore, in discussing Rwanda, an implicit comparison is made with Burundi. Here, the designation of the Burundian conflict as a long-term low-intensity process with episodic intensity locates people in this process in a particular way. It seems to suggest that refugees left the country in early 1990s for the camps in northwestern Tanzania, but it fails to account for the dynamic relations between these camps and Burundi and other conflicts in the region.

This simple construction of the conflict in Burundi misrepresents the nature of the conflict and the way conflict was experienced by diverse groups of people in Burundi. There are two problems here: (i) the review does not seem to think about the nature of conflict from a HIV/AIDS perspective to see what the interactions might be; (ii) Burundi is analysed in relation to the overall purpose of the review rather than looking at its specific conflict context to engage with the experiences of people and the characteristics of HIV related to that experience. As discussed above, this is the function of the methodological orientation of the review. In its comparative format, it chooses to focus on a set of general mechanisms that are considered as significant in revealing the possibility of a general relationship between conflict and HIV/AIDS.

The review seems to have a generic understanding of conflict which is determined according to the intensity of violence, the kind of displacement that is observed, and the nature of armed groups participating. This framing view informs the interpretation of the Burundian conflict as low-intensity and episodically violent. However, it is not clear why this way of thinking about conflict, and how this classifies the Burundian conflict is relevant to think about the intersection between conflict and HIV/AIDS. If the conditions under which HIV spreads are taken to be the determining factor for understanding various intersections between the conflict and HIV in people's lives, then the discussion could be very different. For example, the earlier chapters revealed that one of the central mechanisms for vulnerability to HIV is linked to gender relations. When these relations are put under pressure because of a conflict, these vulnerabilities are exacerbated. The long conflict in Burundi means that many people were dislocated more than once and they had to move within the country and between Burundi and a number of neighboring countries, such as the DRC and Tanzania. Furthermore, people who were armed and joined the rebellion were also moving within the country and between the country and its neighbors. This mobility combined with the separation of many men and women from each other leading to a break down in their families meant that gender vulnerabilities were stretched to their limits. Under the conflict circumstances, gender vulnerabilities were transformed into a new set of risks for HIV. The duration of the conflict was long enough to create a social space for these new risks to become generalized across the country. In addition to these circumstances, the overall conflict context and its duration meant that large parts of the country were inaccessible to HIV/AIDS sensitization and to prevention-based interventions that were rolled out in other places across Africa. From this perspective, the nature of the Burundian conflict is highly relevant for the consideration of risks to HIV spread. Not considering these conditions, obscures the role of mechanisms such as gender in the creation of further risks to HIV during conflict.

The Burundian case should have been analysed in aspects that are relevant for HIV/AIDS consideration in its own specific instances. In the absence of this, what we have as the picture of conflict and HIV in the review is that of *Burundi light*. In attempting to see the evidence from a general point of view, the review misses particular experiences which might have much to say on this relationship. By not paying attention to contextual knowledge the review is (a) not thinking about relevant policies for those who live in conflict contexts; (b) undermining the effectiveness of policies targeting people in conflict contexts; and (c) raising ethical questions about policies targeting people without paying attention to their lived experiences of conflict and HIV/AIDS.

The next section focuses on the kind of data excluded by the selection criteria used in the review. Burundians are being silenced by the review and more generally by the international approach to HIV/AIDS and security. Thus, the section presents knowledge that is precluded from the review. In this process, the aim is to engage with other causal stories that are available to engage with the causal story that is considered as more relevant by the review.

Burundians' Burundi

The material presented in the earlier chapters, highlighting the complex intersections of conflict and HIV/AIDS in people's lives in Burundi, presents an existing understanding of the circumstances within which HIV/AIDS is experienced. Furthermore, it reflects how people who experienced the conflict consider the existence and importance of the relationship between the conflict and HIV/AIDS. The aim in this section, by providing a close look at the issues raised in the chapters, is to highlight the kind of mechanisms that are observed in these reflections in relation to the conflict and HIV/AIDS. This is relevant: (a) to understand the content of the relationship between conflict and HIV/AIDS beyond the limited framing provided by the review; and (b) to consider why these provide an evidential basis to engage with the discussion. People's reflections on their experiences present a picture that is much more complex and varied than the one framed by the above-discussed review. The interviews present multiple causal stories that give content to the mechanisms that are relevant to the relationship between conflict and HIV/AIDS. The multiple stories reflect people's varied positions both during and after the conflict in relation to changing social relations. These locate concerns about HIV/AIDS in Burundi into a number of dynamic process that have influenced people, in particular, women's lives throughout the conflict.

In the previous chapters one of the most striking concerns according to many interviewees was the issue of mobility during the long conflict. These concerns were presented in multiple forms underwriting differentiated and yet parallel processes in people's lives. In contrast, the review considers this intense rearrangement of population and people's lives as a relationship between urban–rural movements. This is then considered as a significant indicator to assess whether there is a relationship between conflict and HIV. Here the assumption is that if there is a link between HIV and conflict, one way of observing this would be to consider the mobility from urban areas where HIV rates were higher to the rural areas where HIV rates were lower at the beginning of the conflict. So the logic is trying to assess how far people from urban areas would have spread the disease into rural areas because of conflict-related dislocation. This is a very simplistic logic. The kinds of mobility patterns that are unpacked present much more complicated processes than the basic urban–rural mobility logic used in the review.

The patterns considered in this book are multilocational and multidirectional compared to the mono-causal mechanisms considered in the review. In addition they are differentiated according to gender, age, and ethnic differences. It is not one or the other of these that is singularly responsible for the risks, but the particular intersections of these that create risks of vulnerability to HIV during conflict. For analytical purposes, one could look at the implications of mobility on the basis of the mobilization patterns of various armed groups and the military. Then, consider the way people's displacement patterns had created diverse patterns of mobility. However, the HIV/AIDS-related concerns for risk are located in the intersection of these dynamic multiple mobility patterns.

People's experiences show that during the conflict many people were dislocated within Burundi and into neighboring countries. People sometimes were dislocated a number of times either from their homes to different places in Burundi or into internally displaced people camps. In other cases they moved out of the country. Some spent time in the Congo and Tanzania at some point during the conflict. The focus on urban–rural movement fails to capture this kind of mobility and also the experiences of repeated dislocations. The impact of repeated displacement is important since, as highlighted by the earlier chapters, this brought a change into Burundian society. The implications of this change are much more complicated than implications assumed in the model of urban–rural logic. The mobility-induced change meant that many more women were moving and were dispersed across the country contrary to their traditional positions in Burundian society. These changes combined with the absence of men in the family meant that women could not easily rely on the protection of traditional patrilineal networks. Over time, this created vulnerabilities for women who were dislocated across the country. Women, as highlighted in the earlier chapters, had to establish multiple relations to survive in the absence of resources. Another aspect of this complexity is the way women's lives intersected with men's mobility. It is clear from the interviews that married women who were able to stay in their communities were also exposed to risks, in particular in relation to vulnerability to HIV, as their husbands might have visited them irregularly during the conflict. This exposed women to the risks their husbands might have been taking with other sexual relationships when outside their communities. In other words, these women might have remained in one place but their husbands' mobility linked them to dispersed sexual networks. While the mobility at multiple levels seems to be one of the mechanisms for risk, its relationship with confinement was also important.

Also, as argued by many women during the interviews, camps both in the country and outside the country created an environment of risk for many women. For instance, some women followed their husbands to Tanzania but once they arrived they were more limited in their movements. For those who were located into internally displaced people camps, their lack of mobility and resources including food meant that they were open to abuse by the soldiers who were supposed to protect them. The mechanism highlighted is about the nature of the camps as confined spaces for those people who cannot protect themselves outside of these camps. Furthermore, they unpack the relationship between the position of the military in relation to these spaces and people who are seeking protection. It presents us with a situation where women were open to exploitation and where the soldiers' attitude towards sex created highly risky conditions for HIV/AIDS. In these spaces the possibility of women's exploitation is linked to HIV spread. This question of protection and security and its relation to sexual abuse is an important mechanism creating new risks for women. Another example is, as discussed in Chapter 3, the coercion methods used by some rebels to persuade girls to join the rebellion clearly played on women's gender vulnerability.

Here it is also important to bring in the implications of the way the military and the armed groups were deployed. As pointed out above, the exposure of more vulnerable women to dynamic military deployment is another important process. Stretched over time this kind of mobility has important implications in creating risks to HIV/AIDS. One of the factors identified in the interviews in relation to men under arms is the time factor influencing their behavior. Two aspects are usually singled out in this: the periods spent away from family and the times spent away from the field to relax. These aspects interact with women's vulnerability in terms of a lack of resources facilitating their availability as sex-workers or for transactional sex. The wealth differential between women and men clearly allowed men to engage with women from a position of power. Women's inability to say "no" to the sexual advances of men were pointed out both by men and women. While men attributed this to the power imbalance in their circumstances due to having arms and more resources, many women reflected on the issue in a more nuanced manner.

The women's reflections also highlight differentiation in women's experiences depending on the spaces where they were able to live and the way these spaces were exposed to the conflict. For women there were survival considerations which made them consider transactional sex or sex-work. They reveal multi-directional processes within which women had to make pragmatic decisions. However, in relation to sexual violence, women did not have any control. Here the discussion identifies a set of mechanisms linked to the mobility of soldiers and armed groups together with changing attitudes towards sex in the long conflict as one of the pathways to increase the risks of the spread of the disease. This unpacking starts to highlight the inadequate framing of these relations in the Spiegel *et al.* review. What is presented in the earlier chapters is a much more complex narrative about people's movements and their reasons for acting in ways through which risks are created.

Reflections on causal relations

The previous two sections considered the experiences of people in Burundi during the conflict. They provided different views on the nature of these experiences and the implications of these for vulnerability to HIV. The last section reflected on the interview material which is presented in the earlier chapters. The interview material provides a complex narrative about the conditions of people during the conflict in Burundi. The Burundi in these reflections is dissimilar to the framing provided in the review by Spiegel and his colleagues. Furthermore, because of the stark dissimilarity, people's reflections naturally lead to a questioning of the assumptions of the review. They question the relevance of the designation of conflict as "low-intensity" and the implications of this for the discussion on conflict and HIV/AIDS. It is clear that this designation neither captures the experiences of civilians nor of soldiers nor of rebels in that context. These experiences also point out that (i) the nature of the conflict and (ii) its duration were significant factors to consider in the relationship between conflict and HIV in Burundi. The divergence here is also a divergence about the modes of knowing. In other words they are two competing claims to knowledge.

In trying to engage with the debate on the relationship between conflict and HIV at the population level, the review constructs a causal model which considers a series of relations as the relevant mechanisms of the location of the conflict—the HIV/AIDS relationship with conflict should it exist. In doing so it focuses on a particular kind of data at the expense of other kinds of data. The mechanisms that are obvious to people in considering the relationship between conflict and HIV are ignored. The mechanisms highlighted in people's reflections not only articulate how conflict and HIV might be related but also and most importantly why and how they might have been linked in the context of Burundi. People's reflections elaborate differentiated and complex causal relations underwriting behavioral mechanisms that are important for HIV/AIDS-related considerations. However, these are missed. In an attempt to create a causal model to consider whether or not the relationship exists at the population level in a comparable form with other countries, the discussion ignores the reasons why it might exist, given, for instance, the gender relations that are under pressure and creating structural vulnerabilities for people. Furthermore, the comparability constraint inevitably required a conceptual reduction to a model relationship between conflict and HIV/AIDS. However, this reduction implies that the review disregards people's experiences within individual countries unless they are a detectable population-based view, which is unlikely given their diversity and complexity.

As the review considers certain relations such as urban–rural mobility at the population level, individuals' mobility patterns and the impact of these patterns on their exposure to violence and HIV disappear from the discussion. Unless there is a statistically significant result in this area they remain hidden. Thus, the significance of different experiences for our understanding of conflict and HIV is lost. Furthermore, as these individual experiences provide causal stories to understand the relationship between conflict, people's vulnerabilities and the disease, once they disappear it becomes harder to understand the mechanisms underlying the assumed to be important relations. In the absence of understanding such mechanisms, the relationship is only considered according to the available infection rates. Another area where this methodological limitation becomes clear relates to sexual violence and rape during the conflict. Again this is considered at the level of populations. When they consider the relationship between rape and HIV they conclude that the data cannot provide significant results at the population level to relate incidents of rape with increased HIV infections.

The considerations on rape reveal why it is that the divergent epistemologies are important. The review's framing of the link between rape and HIV spread in conflict significantly diverges from the experiences of people in Burundi. This is due to two interrelated reductions: (i) by considering the Burundian case as a *long-term low-intensity* conflict the scale of sexual violence is implicitly considered to be less of an issue. Here the comparison is with Rwandan genocide. They take this case as significant to consider, as a benchmark, for arriving at their conclusion: (ii) the significance criteria they have on rape is based on the statistical significance of those acts being reported and the correlation between such reporting and the incidents of HIV in the large surveys that are included in the review. Our interviews point out that many incidents of rape are experienced by women under various circumstances. From their point of view, rape was significant to their lives both during and after the conflict. The significance here is framed according to people's livelihood needs and their considerations of risks for HIV underwriting their wellbeing considerations. Also important in the interviews was the way this issue was brought up by women who were victims and by men who were perpetrators or witnesses to these acts. These were reported independently of each other time and again. Given this, it is hard to ignore the significance of these events in informing risks and vulnerabilities to HIV. The issue of rape is an important concern not only because it might lead to an actual infection, but also because it creates conditions for people to be vulnerable in the long-term to HIV and to other social problems. The focus on population-wide effects not only means that people's lives are not considered in their context but also the knowledge embedded in their experiences and how this may affect subsequent behavior is ignored. People's reflections on their experiences during the conflict reveal mechanisms that create conditions and allow women to be exploited in a given context. Yet, they are disqualified from providing knowledge to a process that will influence the policies targeting them. Does this lead to a problem of misrecognition of the needs and demands of people in particular contexts?

From a HIV/AIDS perspective the particular approach to knowledge evident in the review has serious implications: (i) the methodology used to assess population-based trends excludes the kinds of contextual knowledge that would reveal the structural vulnerabilities that create sexual violence; (ii) the inability to engage with people's experiences leads to taking the technical inability to connect rape with HIV as representative; (iii) this takes non-reporting as an absence but ignoring reasons behind people's reluctance to participate in particular kinds of data collection. On the whole, the distorted significance attributed to certain kinds of knowledge, i.e., those correlated with infection or incidence rates, creates a shortsighted situation. For a process or particular mechanism to have significance for HIV/AIDS concerns *it does not have to be considered only in relation to infection and incidence rates.* Although these measures are important to consider for understanding the general situation, they are *post facto* measures to consider what has happened but they don't explain why what is observed has happened. Therefore, to understand the possible relationship between conflict and HIV/AIDS their use as a measure of assessment is going to provide a blunt instrument at best.

The methodological commitment brought out here highlights an important problem described by Brian Wynne as "the institutional neglect of issues of public meaning and the presumptive imposition of such meaning (and identities) on those publics and the public domain" (2002: 402). This view on neglect identifies not only a gap between the way security and HIV/AIDS are considered independent of the views and concerns of people in Burundi thinking about conflict and HIV, it also points out an embedded and systematized process of sidelining people's needs and views within the international policy fora. This is linked to decisions on the questions that are considered to be relevant. The methodological position in the review constructs a way of thinking and asking questions about conflict. In this, the meaning of conflict in Burundi is inferred without a link to the way people in Burundi reflect on the conflict. The relevance of the questions that matter to international policy processes assumes and attributes relevance of these to people as a generic category. While it is clear that the methodology used in the review structurally excludes voices, the choice of this methodological framework indicates a pre-methodological decision on what matters in this field. In this process the experts' views attribute a particular meaning to conflict and HIV independent of the people's experiences.

Undoubtedly expert knowledge has its relevance, but as Wynne argues "its salience, validity and authority with respect to a public issue are still conditional" (2002: 403). Here the experts' position vis-à-vis the public is important. The public are located as the ground on which the conditions of validity and salience of expert knowledge should be considered. The expert decision to prioritize one method over another in a given field is also linked to Longino's discussions of background beliefs. These beliefs not only inform the content of the hypothesis but they also represent a commitment to a particular way of knowing. This commitment disqualifies people's experiences and their reflections as relevant for obtaining knowledge. Arguably, this is based on a distinction between cognition based on "scientifically determined" ways of knowing and the way people acquire knowledge through experience. Mary S. Morgan questions this delineation when she argues that:

> the fact that everyone lives in a society and knows something of it, means that the facts about events and relationships drawn from personal experience cannot simply be dismissed as ignorance just because they are not known through the methods of science.
>
> (Morgan 2008: 21)

In short, people know their context as they interact with each other and with that context.

If one agrees with Wynne on the conditionality of expert knowledge, one also needs to consider how this conditionality needs to be discussed. Could one discuss conditionality only on the basis of how particular knowledge relates to a hypothesis? Or, should it be discussed in the way expert knowledge limits the kind of knowledge that is seen as relevant. If we are interested in the link between conflict and HIV/AIDS, is the conditionality a function of the lack of epidemiological research and other survey-based data or is it about the expert frame that fixes the discussion at the level of data collection at the expense of knowledge embedded in people's experiences? Critically, the former reduces the debate to a technical discussion of knowledge without questioning whether the kind of knowledge we are looking for in this way will reveal the mechanisms that are relevant for thinking about conflict and HIV/AIDS. Engaging with the former question, i.e., on the lack of epidemiological data and research, will not change the approach and lead to engaging with people's experiences since the parameters of the discussion will remain fixed to the population-level concerns.

The issue here is not only about the nature of conflict and the way the questions posed by international policy experts (including academic researchers) frame the debate. It is also about what we think policy makers need to know about HIV/AIDS for the development of policies targeting people's lives. It is here that institutional interests and perspectives on the nature of knowledge become important in framing what needs to be known about the problem. As I have argued, the international policy approach has focused on population-wide assessments and measures to engage, prioritize, and develop interventions. Population-wide indicators signal the severity of the problem and the need for intervention. Yet, most policy interventions attempt to influence the way people act in their everyday lives. For many, if not most, interventions on social and behavior change to reduce risks it matters whether these policies are based on knowledge that is related to the cognitive world of those who are targeted. As Justine O. Parkhurst argues, it is important to understand that people don't simply change behavior only because of "specific interventions, [but] rather than from a combination of multiple interrelated and combined factors, of which any intervention will only be a part" (2008: 281). It is therefore imperative to understand how these interrelated and combined factors interact in people's everyday lives and the basis on which people act in such a context (Seckinelgin 2008). If one of the central aims of the policy interventions in HIV/AIDS is to alter behavior for preventative outcomes, then unless people's knowledge of themselves in context are considered as a key part of the knowledge of HIV/AIDS in context, most of these policy interventions will have limited use. This move also requires a switch in what is assumed to be the position of people's knowledge based on their own experiences in relation to the more technically verified and constructed scientific knowledge of the disease. According to Wynne knowing "a particular situation or condition held by such individuals and groups is often 'more specifically accurate' about that problem even while 'less generally authorative' than the knowledge held by professional scientist" (Wynne 1991 in Morgan 2008: 23).

Conclusion

This chapter has considered the difference between two sets of knowledge claims: the expert knowledge claims on security and HIV/AIDS that was embodied in the systematic review discussed in the last chapter and the knowledge claims related to people's experiences reported throughout this book. I used the way expert knowledge frames both the Burundian conflict and its relationship to HIV/AIDS as an analytical entry point to unpack knowledge claims and their sources. I then discussed the implications of these claims. Here the specific HIV/AIDS-related needs in relation to the Burundian conflict are the grounds for this discussion. The experiences considered earlier in the book demonstrate that the conflict was complex and traumatic for many people in Burundi. For instance, for many people the conflict's duration and intensity was different and contrary to its designation in the review.

The considerations in the chapter are about the nature of evidence required to understand people's experiences if the policy is to successfully address their needs. It is argued that the kind of methodological commitments evident in the review to extract information and to assess the existence of a relationship exclude people's experience-based knowledge. Their orientation is based on expert background beliefs on the nature of the relationship between people and HIV/AIDS in conflict, what is important for people, and the kind of data that is required to develop policies. The challenge I identified for this approach is that people's voices and experiences are removed from the process. The end product has little reliance on people's experiences and their needs which are linked to those experiences. For instance, from the HIV/AIDS perspective the lack of gender concern in a systematic way goes against the way people's experiences were gendered in a context-specific manner.

The sources of background beliefs/assumptions that frame knowledge claims as evidence and lead to policy prescriptions matter. The expert knowledge on how a policy should work might be correct in the abstract, but as Wynne puts it, the relevance of such knowledge is conditional on the way people's experiences reflect on these issues. Furthermore, the degree to which people's experiences inform the experts' claims provides a way to think about this conditionality. This position also raises important questions about the knowledge claims within international policy debates on HIV/AIDS in which the security and HIV/AIDS approach has become an important area. It also prompts an idea about what is the aim of the claims underwriting this approach if it has little link to people's experiences.

The chapter ends by pointing out the importance of people's knowledge of their own experiences and conditions. I argued that the way of knowing in these experiences might be different from obtaining knowledge through scientific techniques, but that this does not make them less relevant. The question one needs to ask of these is not about their technical competence but their relevance for HIV/AIDS concerns of people in particular contexts. The chapter argues that people's knowledge needs to provide the underlying assumptions for understanding the conflict and HIV/AIDS relationship as it relates to their lives.

8 Communities of policy and communities of everyday life

This chapter discusses the way people dynamically engage with HIV/AIDS to influence their own lives. It also considers that while dealing with their own problems people influence other's lives in Burundi. In this way it also contributes to the epistemological discussion of the last chapter by analysing how people think about their community activity. There are also three other reasons to include this chapter here. First, to consider the ways in which people engage with HIV/AIDS in different ways, including the creation of new associations or sensitization processes led by individuals within communities. Second, to look at people's narratives about their motivations to create groups and associations which indicate that when ex-combatants came back, many communities already had an understanding of HIV/AIDS. Third, it is to emphasize the importance of local agency in dealing with HIV/AIDS.

While it is true that the intersection of conflict and HIV/AIDS pressurized and created various gender-based vulnerabilities to HIV, people in Burundi dynamically engage with the disease and its causes. The aim of this chapter is to provide a grounded understanding of the ways in which people exercise their agency in this context. People's narratives highlight instances and processes that are not very well understood by the top-down policy processes that often derive from international policy contexts that are "unable to respond to local realities and treating beneficiaries as passive" (Gibbs 2010: 1621; also see Campbell 2003; Gruber and Caffrey 2005; Gregson *et al.* 2007). The narratives that are reported below indicate social relations that are the outcomes of actors' engagement with their lives at times of conflict and HIV/AIDS. In these narratives, social relations create transformative spaces and processes that address a number of the pressing problems people face (Campbell and Cornish 2010: 1573). The spaces created by these groups indicate a process of confidence building that also underwrites the safety of those revealing their HIV status (Vaughan 2010). Here what is important is the way people deal with questions of behavior change "that are realistic within the constraints of their everyday lives" and allowing them to "discuss ways in which they might challenge unhealthy social relations" (Campbell and Cornish 2010: 1573). It is also worth emphasizing that these processes reveal the contours of social change that are initiated by people's agency deployed to deal with their problems within their communities.

Interestingly, many of these narratives reveal that—contrary to the assumed silence of women—it is the women with HIV who become the driving force behind community groups. It is also revealing that they are able to talk about their HIV status within their groups to influence others' behavior. Here the agency of women is deployed in a similar way to our observations throughout the research experience when contrary to the assumed silence of women, they were very keen to tell their stories. It is through this story-telling that they hope to influence social change. Here the community activity and the groups they create form the space within which women are able to talk about their experiences. Many of these groups are not formed singularly to deal with HIV/AIDS-related issues; instead, they are attempts to deal with complicated needs of people in their everyday lives. They deal with people's material needs such as helping them to pull together their resources to farm. Considering the period when these groups emerged through the late 1990s and early 2000s, they are also attempts to maintain and strengthen communities impacted by the conflict. The conflict made women more vulnerable, as their male relatives were often involved in the conflict and away. These community initiatives are attempts by women to pull together their resources and deal with their problems. These avenues of community activity provide ways of influencing social norms, such as the gender governance, in the country. They provide spaces and processes through which women implicitly negotiate social change due to their experiences of HIV/AIDS and conflict (Campbell and Cornish 2010: 1574–75). Here the process is subtle and based on complex interactive processes in the socio-cultural context within which people live.

Different ways to influence social change

M1 was part of a team that worked with the DDR program and was a journalist before this. We interviewed him to hear about his DDR experience and his motivations to create a community association in his commune called *Ndababurire-SIDA* (Let me warn you about HIV/AIDS). This association was created in 2000 and formally registered as a community association in 2002. At the time of the interview the association was receiving funding from CNLS through CPLS under the Ministry of AIDS. The funding was part of the requirement by the Global Fund and the World Bank to include community and civil society groups for providing funds to the country. M1 said that he began to think about the association in 1999. The association had two founding members and gradually 30 others joined them.

M1: On my hillside, there was a widower he married again to a Rwandese woman in 1989. He worked in Bujumbura. In the neighborhood, there was a rich young man who used go to Bujumbura for business. He used to buy things in Bujumbura and sell them in Bujumbura Rural. The young man had an affair with the young Rwandese woman. The young man also had an elder brother who was said to be sterile as his wife had no children. The same young man had an ongoing affair with his brother's wife too. The young man must have been infected with HIV somewhere in Bujumbura. He therefore infected the two women. Those two women then contaminated their husbands. Now all those people are dead. You see, men go to Bujumbura and go to sex-workers. They come back home and contaminate their wives. And you may know also that women transmitted the virus to other two men who were temporally hired by them to work on their fields. Now, 30 families have been infected, and most of them are dead. This is a real story. That chain, I know, I think all 30 AIDS related dead came from that one young man. The young man dies in 1992, the two men died in 1995 and the two women died in 1997. The young sister of the young man was a student; she died of AIDS too. We don't know exactly when and how she was infected. I was aware of all these dead since 1990 and wanted to help and contribute to the HIV awareness and fight it.

INTERVIEWER: Could you please tell us more about people's perceptions of HIV/AIDS?

MI: They think that people get thin, this issue becomes part of peoples' conversations, this talk is always there, they talk about it when they drink, eat and work with others. They don't talk about tuberculosis in the same way, HIV+ people are isolated and some say they are HIV+ to get help. In where we are in Bujumbura Rural it is hard for HIV+ to say publically about their status. In Bujumbura as the help is more available they say they are HIV+. There was a teacher in the local Lycée and who was very ill in 1999, we needed to hold him to get him out of his bed. He was only helped by an expat to get ARVs, now he is OK. Before it was even harder when someone was ill, the community did not want to help. They said he is a teacher he can contaminate others. So if someone suffers from this he does not have a place in the community. He needs to go to an urban center.

INTERVIEWER: How about ARVs, do people have access to them here?

MI: There are no ARVs, only in Bujumbura, and only for those who know how to get them.

SPEAKER: Do you get tested outside Bujumbura?

MI: Many did not want to be tested in their communities and have to come to Bujumbura. They did not want their community to know their status so going somewhere else was important. If someone is not well, it is like other diseases, you need treatment. If you are HIV+, how will you get help if you test privately and away from your home?—If you don't get help—cannot get help, then you do not want to test. So poverty, distance to testing and fear for the future stop people testing. HIV is not curable if you have it you will die-our association is sensitizing that HIV/AIDS does not mean dead. A problem is that people don't want to know their status, how do we change this mentality. Many people still do not want to hear about testing.

We think that the government has been weak in relation to the donors. It was not able to push donors and get them support the necessity to continue sensitization. We have a largely illiterate population. We have to develop alternative and effective sensitization methods in order to have effective results. Plays can be one of these methods. Between 2004–2006 we were doing lots of sensitization and HIV awareness was growing in the communities. But we saw that this diminishes when sensitization slows down. Our idea in our project was to have 5000 people well trained on sensitization and prevention. When we began public sensitization in hillsides, we saw sometimes 800 people were coming to participate. But then there were others saying to these people that "if you are participating in these sessions, may be it is because you are HIV+. Or you must be getting money for this."

There was no sensitization during the war for either soldiers in the military or the rebels. Now after the war it has stopped in the hillsides and they have missed sensitization altogether. The areas most at risk are the semi-rural areas because donors with mass sensitization are in large urban areas but not outside areas such as Bujumbura Rural, there is only one health center here. When I was working with an international radio group, I produced a report on sex-workers in Buyenzi. They only accepted men with condoms. Outside the town, women accepted without condoms for lots of money. My analysis is that sensitization is low in semi-rural areas and high in urban areas.

Our approach is to get larger communities to participate, we needed to promote local associations (as many INGOs could not go to these communities due to the security issues), find money to help sensitization activity and build common projects. This integrated approach tries to include a HIV/AIDS component in different projects in order to take into account people's mentality, their needs and their interests to get jobs. For example, we wanted to fund youth groups to make films on different issues related with HIV/AIDS and to show these to other young people and to the communities. Once in 2006 we showed a film like that, we asked young people what they thought of the film. I saw emotions, 10 minute silence; they were touched by the film.

INTERVIEWER: Could you please tell us more about your work?

M1:   We collaborate with other organizations; we worked with Jesuit Relief Services. They agreed to give training for six months to 10 members of our association on HIV prevention, modes of transmission, how to provide psycho-social support and they also trained others who went to the hillsides to sensitize. We targeted hardest hit areas and went to the churches after mass to give sensitization. Those people [members] who have positions in communities, teachers, nurses and others, target groups they work with to maximize the impact of sensitization. In 2002–2005 we targeted 15,000 people. In 2002–2003 people did not really come to us. We thought we had to change our methods, so started to show films on HIV prevention and how it is to live as a HIV+ person. Then came our work with JRS. Young people liked and were interested in films. So as a method of sensitization it

worked. Showing films is appropriate but it is hard in areas with no elec-
tricity. The idea is to insert HIV/AIDS in projects-like into sports or income
generating activities. This will increase impact. It is easier for people to
accept the message and to understand people who would never come only
for HIV sensitization.

These reflections provide interesting insights about the way people reacted to
the appearance of HIV/AIDS in their community. In reflecting on the time
line of the disease in his community M1's insights are about the complex
processes that inform people's behavior in relation to the disease. Part of this
behavior is about the local dynamics in relation to illness. This is also condi-
tioned by another important part of their behavior, stigma. M1's interview
sheds light on the issue of stigma attached to the disease. In this particular
community people were talking about HIV/AIDS; however, the lack of
material, social, and conceptual resources created rhetoric aimed at distancing the problem, wish it away, from the individuals and from their close
environment. The relationship between people's overall concerns about their
future and the way they engage with the disease was linked. Even if they had
wanted to be tested they prefer to be tested away from their communities.
This allowed them to control the way they engage with their own HIV status.
The absence of socio-cultural resources to deal with HIV+ status creates
greater caution on whether to reveal one's status. It is then that M1's association came in as a mechanism to deal with some of these resource problems.
M1's reflections also highlight the kind of community work that is productive
in this area. Work that aims to address the overall context of vulnerability
seems to allow people to engage with HIV/AIDS issues as a part of the
broader context without being singled out on the basis of their health status.
It is also clear from the discussion that their initial work based within their
own community is being scaled up to deal with problems of the disease in a
much wider society. This is indicated by the way they received funding from
the central HIV/AIDS budget through CNLS. This raises the question how
they maintain their link within their community while also stretching out. It
also raises an interesting issue on the relationship between mass sensitizations
and micro-community work led by those who are respected in their communities. The issue is the gap between the provision of information and trans-
lating this into relevant knowledge for behavior change. The provision of
generalized medical and behavioral information requiring people to change
their lives creates anxiety. If this is not handled sensitively it could transform
trusting relations in a community into relations of distrust. The community
group here acts as an important conduit to translate this medical and behavioral model coming from top-down policy frameworks to effective local
policy intervention. In doing this work it also creates a space within which the
digestion and adaptation of this information to locally relevant ways of
engaging with the disease could take place. The importance of individuals in
expanding this space is an important part of the community work. The next

interview and the focus group extracts turn to this issue. Before looking at these it is also important to emphasize that M1's discussion of the HIV/AIDS knowledge among ex-combatants is important. It shows that, in the context of the conflict, ex-combatants lacked information.

While role models are important to influence people's behavior in a community, the agency required for this depends on those who feel that they can talk about their status within their communities. This is a challenging task. N1 was 42 and living in a commune of Ngozi province with her two children; she had lost her third child and her husband had died in 2000. She was HIV+ and a member of various organizations and associations; she worked as an *aide infirmière* (nurse assistant) at the health center.

N1: I live with my two children, one is in the lycée and the other is in the primary school. I am HIV+ and people know that. I am the first to talk about my status in the commune. It was initially not easy, some said that I don't want to be with men that this was my way of refusing men. Also, in my job, colleagues said that I am not ill, not HIV+, that I just want money. I was among the first group to get CD4 count [among a group of 20], around 2002. At the time we already had CPLS Ngozi, CNLS invited us [HIV+] to a seminar, I was working at Ngozi hospital at the time. It was for seven days, we received a certificate. We were 40 invited and all openly HIV+. At the time, there were no more than 40 openly HIV+ in the province. They told us to teach others, not to hide, that being together makes people strong, that changing the mood of HIV, helping others to come forward will help change health. Then maybe in 2003 I came here [health center] to work on December 1st [the World Aids Day] I asked the communal administrator if I could talk about my status openly. He said yes. I used to be invited to this event after this but now—no. People are not informed the new communal administrator does not even know we exist. Maybe she does not like us, she does not even want to see us. There are 35 now accepting their HIV+ status (only seven are men).

INTERVIEWER: What do you think about the stigma?

N1: We are discriminated against. I had been working for two years when I found out I was HIV+. Now many at the health center refuse that I give the injections. One woman in an open meeting said that she does not want me to give injections. There was another man who supported her. The communal administrator was chairing the meeting, and I asked to speak. And she refused. She said publicly that I am no longer able to give injections. It has been two years. So you must understand that we are discriminated against by the administrative authority. They also allow others to discriminate against us. People say I lied when I said I was HIV+ and that if I were HIV+ then I should been dead as there was another nurse who died of the disease. I am still alive so I cannot be HIV+. Many people say to visitors, if you go to her, you will be dead. Here some accept to use your glass but there is still discrimination. In 2003 when I was ill no one came to visit me.

INTERVIEWER: How do you help others?

N1:   We [her association] have regular meetings for the committee members and they pay their own transport fees. Here people are really poor, I cannot tell you. Before, I had an account with the cooperative bank people could not contribute, for two years there were no contributions. During those two years I was replaced as I was ill. The person that replaced me was not active. They had elections she was not reelected. I was voted in three months [August] ago. The first general meeting was on October 25th, 22 out of 35 people came. We support each other. For example on October 25th we had a problem. One HIV+ woman member lives with a man, they are not officially married, they have two kids. He moved in with another woman. He took everything so during the meeting we asked all members to give something (plate, a cup, anything) and on December 10th in our next meeting we will give these to her. We have also another woman who is a widow, on one of the hillsides, her house was destroyed and we'll help her re-build it. Some will do the work as they don't have money to contribute. Now the widow lives in a small house. Also in 2005 when my child died and I was ill, they helped me. They worked on my land, they planted potatoes. We encouraged people to join our group, many women did.

This interview highlights the socio-cultural context within which N1 exercised her agency and how her agency interacted with existing attitudes and pre-judices. Furthermore, her situation represents how at times it is difficult to engage with the disease even in a local medical context. The medical context here was one of the communities she belonged too. This was framed within the workspace. An interesting issue here is the way in which she, by being open about her status, was negotiating with others on attitudes and behavior in the context of HIV/AIDS. Her narrative also shows that this medical con-text was located in the larger context of the community, as the community administrator was deciding on her professional activity. Another community was a group of people who had got together to help each other, and most were HIV+. This group represented those people who were discriminated against in the larger community. However, the work they did clearly was not hidden from the others. Considering that they expanded their membership to 35 shows that the implicit negotiation with their community was a dynamic process and represented a changing nature of community attitudes. However, it also shows her determination to be open about her status and to organize a group in her commune to deal with the stigma. In this the impact of their work was undoubtedly important as it went beyond dealing with stigma to dealing with people's material needs.

It is also interesting to look at a community group which was not founded to deal with HIV/AIDS but to focus on material needs during the conflict. In Gitega province at a group discussion with a local association, 19 members had joined the meeting. There were only two men present. One was 43 and married with three children and the other was 44 and married with four children. The age of the women varied from 18 to 43 years; the youngest two did not have children but the others did. The association's name was *Twi-nyungunyanye* (Let's Come Together). The main aim of the association was to take care of plants and to work together on the land.

O1:   We began thinking about how to come together and build an association. We then came together and began cultivating vegetables in 2000. The harvest was good. Then we rented some land for another season. You know I am HIV+. Since I know, I live well with the virus. I joined this association [local branch of a larger NGO] in 2001 this NGO gave us seeds and fertilizers. We are happy at this stage. In the beginning we were 15 and now we have 20 people. When we plant vegetables we help each other. We give some money to each other for health care. If one has no strength for the work others will take over and do the work for him/her on the common land. We also go to his/her field together once a week to help. We don't want help from outside forever. Two years ago we opened an account at the cooperative bank in Gitega. If one needs money for school fees or his/her child is ill we borrow money from our account and we reimburse it after. Three members of our association are HIV+.

INTERVIEWER: How do they fit in ?

O1:   There is no discrimination. Even if some of us are ill, no one complains. It is a good sign that others join us. While working together, we talk about HIV/AIDS. Some went for testing. If the results are negative they are happy. It gives them the strength to keep working hard.

P1:   Those who are HIV+ teach us well. We appreciate it.

R1:   At the beginning the objective was that those who are HIV+ would teach us so we are informed and think to protect ourselves.

Q1:   She [head of the association] came to us and told that: "I am HIV+." We said: "No. Those who are AIDS, they are ill, they are dead and we see that you are a healthy woman." We thought that all HIV+ people were ill. Now we know the reality. We can talk, laugh and work together with no problem.

S1:   So we started to work together to build the association. This association helps us to be strong, to stay strong and to act responsibly. No one here would run after bright and shining things that could get us into trouble. We cultivate our land, we have life, and we see our future is good. Association is good. It allows us to give advice to other sisters.

Q1:   At the beginning really we did not believe she was HIV+. She helped us to change the image of HIV+ people. You know Uwufise urumuri ntahakurira hasi [the one who has the torch will not put the cassava bread on the ground]. You go gently to her you can go with questions and she answers them. It is helpful. It keeps you centered so you are not going for bright things. We did not know about HIV+ or HIV–. She insisted gently telling us to go for testing. She said that "you see me, I thought I had different illnesses. I came to know my real situation after testing. Now I know and I can plan."

TI: For us, for example for me, I am 32 with two children and no husband, I am a young widow. Sometimes you are lonely. The association helps me ... I have people to talk to. We cultivate, so we have some money and it gives strength to go on.

OI: Amongst women and men, it is easy. When we work, we talk. It is good. We exchange ideas among men and women. At the beginning it was slow and then people progressively opened up. Slowly, we go to others, especially to young. Now we have five young girls and four young men. We keep advising them. We began to talk among women we encouraged each other to go to test. Then some men slowly came in and went for test and they convinced other men to go for testing. Now it is time for the young.

UI: We who are HIV+, we used to share our experience with others and we use to give them advice. We tell people to take care and to organize their life.

QI: At the beginning it was tough. It was very difficult. As women ... , the process required us to gather all my courage, to stand and give testimony of my life. When I did once, I felt I could continue ... so some men listened to me. At times men I talked to don't listen but I know they will remember things I say.

VI: For us men, those who are HIV+, those women, they are strong. They talked to us, and it was hard for them. They taught us well. We appreciate their efforts.

INTERVIEWER: Do people change their behavior?

VI: Now, there is a strong message against sexual relations outside marriage. People behaved irresponsibly. Things are getting better now. People know now that HIV/AIDS can kill. Community facilitators are also here, they come to teach people during public meetings. At the beginning people thought HIV/AIDS was like other illness. They thought it was not a serious matter.

XI: Even to those who do not listen, we give advice. We just tell them Agasozi kari k-intahanurwa kahiye abagabo babona [the hill which never gets advice burnt without any help from people around]. Men want to involve with women in inappropriate sexual relations. They know we love them and they know we are right and trying to help. Now we are happy that there is sensitization on HIV/AIDS at school. So kids come home with some information on HIV/AIDS in their notebooks. This gives an opening to talk about HIV/AIDS. They are also curious and asking questions. Because this started at school it is a good thing. They listen better this way when we talk about it. Also we talk about flirting, courting and other things with them. We tell them, especially to girls that, if someone gives money or other nice things it might be dangerous and they must leave the situation.

The discussion in this group presents an interesting process in which resource shortages and needs brought a number of people together. There were a number of HIV+ people within the group. Here the discussion highlights two levels of discrimination. The discrimination they talk about refers to the social relations impacting women's lives during the conflict. For some, it was the problem of being a widow and not having access to resources which made them join the group. There is also the discrimination linked with the disease. However, the HIV/AIDS was not the primary motivation for the group's formation. Those who were HIV+ talked about their status openly within the group—the way made possible from the trust that had been built among the members by working together. The process of engaging with HIV/AIDS was diffused in their work in general. This seems to have allowed HIV+ members to talk about their experiences without overwhelming others and have allowed others to have a space to digest the information and also to observe the experiences of HIV+ members. In other words, the group created its own common experiences of the disease in context. In this process gender norms and their implications were also discussed.

The attitude change towards more openness and its associated behavior also influenced the way the group engaged with others in their community. Their internal experiences encouraged them to talk about HIV to others too. In other words they felt this was the right thing to do, X1 says, "even to those who do not listen." Her point here is that it is important to allow a different language and discourse to emerge in the community in relation to sex and sexual relations to influence HIV/AIDS risks. Another important point is the way V1 talks about his relationship with women who were talking about HIV. The discussion reveals that gender norms regulating social relations and forms of masculinity in particular were identified as important issues for risks to HIV/AIDS. From this identification the group moved towards a dynamic renegotiation of gender norms through the micro-processes they described such as just talking in the fields or talking about their experiences with others with the implicit aim to change behavior. The beginning of this renegotiation was linked to the symbolic impact of women acting on their own to talk about their own experiences within the community. This process has allowed a space for discussion to emerge. In this the authority to speak was a function of the experience of the disease and it is encouraged by their experiences within their community group.

In the discussions we had with them the group also highlighted some important tensions in relation to the post-conflict context. When asked about the conflict and their reflections on the way it interacted with HIV/AIDS, there was an initial silence and N1 said that "the war is over now. We are hoping that it will never return." After another pause they all said that "HIV/AIDS is a war."

X1: People were fleeing. Women were assaulted because they were defenseless and poor. You were in the bush, you felt like you were dying. If you needed food you did what you did … Men came from the bush entered into your house during the night. They came to rape people.

V1: There is still an issue with IDPs. Ethnic divide is an issue but there is also hunger. They used to produce food in their land, but during the war they could not. The situation is different in each hillside. Here some people fled, some did not. We tried to protect their belongings. We want them to come back to cultivate their land. They say they fear people might kill them.

The tensions discussed here show the difficulty for those who left their communities to come back. In this particular community the aim is to move beyond the problems experienced during the conflict. This attitude developed through their common effort to deal with their problems within their community. In other words, this work resulted in new relations and new ways of thinking about living together.

However, these were not available to those people who had left during the conflict and for those who had joined the rebellion or the military. These groups did not have social spaces that would allow them to develop these attitudes. Critically the DDR process also did not create such a space. Another important point here is the size of the community seems to make people understand each other in a different way. When X1 is talking about people being raped in their community, the way she talks about it indicates that she knew these people at the time of these events. In other words, there is a certain transparency to the relations which forms a common view on the past and their experiences. Where such communal links are not as strong these experiences might become much more discriminatory. This is highlighted in the following discussion.

In a discussion with the members of an association in a Bujumbura commune, 15 members participated in the meeting. The age group ranged from 17 to 70 years and included both men and women who had children. There were also many widows in the association. One of the founders of the association began the discussion by explaining the motivation behind the association.

> After the war broke out there were many difficulties, one was HIV/AIDS. With a friend, we were committed to help, we had friends who died of HIV. We thought of an association to sensitize and protect people. HIV kills and increases poverty. We created the association in 2001 in this commune, but we also wanted to reach others in the city. The main objectives were to fight HIV and poverty. We have trained some trainers both here and elsewhere in Bujumbura. We see poverty and we are trying to now find projects to help families, especially orphans. Although we are not a big association we are still helping people. We gave chemical and organic fertilizers, we see people who are engaged in the fields, now they need houses, schools, clothing many people need support. We are 13 people visiting beneficiaries. We hope for more support for lasting development, especially for the youth.

After this introduction their member/beneficiaries joined the discussion and talked about their experiences to the association. W1 was a widowed woman of 60 with six children and also looking after one grandchild whose father had died of AIDS. She said that:

> We are happy to see good relations come to us, they asked us how many orphans we have and promised us seeds and fertilizers so we could

cultivate land, have food, seeds for the next season. We are now preparing land for the next season. We are all widows and have orphans. There are benefits to being together.

When asked what they thought about HIV/AIDS, a large number of participants responded that "(HIV) is why we are widows." It was also clear from the discussion that the association was active in engaging its members in HIV/AIDS sensitization activities as a part of their overall work. A common view expressed was the fact that *everyone was trained* and they all participate in sensitization meetings and promote testing. Furthermore, they mentioned that *they accept visits at home.* This is an important indication of the way the association managed over time to overcome an important stigma attached to HIV/AIDS. However, linked to stigmatization this particular issue of home visits has a complicated pattern, differing according to the social space within which such visits are conducted. We had a more nuanced view of this issue, for instance, in a separate discussion with Y1. She was the coordinator of a country-wide NGO in Bujumbura and organized home visits to their beneficiaries across the urban space.

Y1:   There is much stigmatization. People tend to point the finger to HIV+ persons. But there I saw some improvement. We visit our beneficiaries at home. We have health specialists in each quartier of the city (Bujumbura) to follow on people and see how they take ARVs. We have our staff: a doctor, nurses and social workers. We also have volunteering members who help and organize visits. In some quartiers such as Buyenzi and Bwiza people asked us not to visit them at home as they see it as stigmatizing. People know us and the say "here they come to visit the HIV+ person." These communities are not sensitized enough, even if they are near to the center of the town. Beneficiaries tell us "don't come to visit us, our landlord would kick us out." But in Cibitoke and Buterere, quartiers that are far from the central Bujumbura there is less discrimination.

This last extract provides further insights to understand how community activity works in a spatially differentiated manner, and the difference between the community work as it has been presented earlier and the professionalized NGO work highlighted in this extract. The NGO here is in a large city (Bujumbura) compared with other community groups working in much smaller communes or in hillsides (*collines*). The NGO functions across various communes in the urban space as it has mostly beneficiaries, rather than members, across this space. The definition of the community for this group does not overlap with a spatial delineation and also members of the NGO do not overlap with the beneficiaries. Therefore, the members of the NGO and their beneficiaries have differentiated relations with the NGO and also with the people living around them. The dynamics of these layered relationships in these differentiated networks complicate the issue of stigma and discrimination emanating from such attitudes. The NGO provides material support through health care, which is undoubtedly a function of both being in the capital and being part of the international aid networks providing resources. This also reliably suggests the professionalization of the relations between the NGO and its beneficiaries. At the same time in order to mediate between these two groups the NGO has volunteers working for them.

Here an interesting more general question is whether the idea of community mobilization as an important process has limits which are, on the one hand, determined by its spatiality and on the other influenced by the degree to which community groups become professionalized organizations dealing with beneficiaries rather than their members (Vielajus and Haeringer 2011). In the above extract from Y1, the reflection suggests that while in the spatiality of an urban space the community group is able to provide services, it is not adding to those beneficiaries an ability to engage within their own immediate social environment.

Agency, mobilization, and community life

This chapter points out a number of important issues for thinking about people's agency and HIV/AIDS interventions in general. Given the conflict context within which the reported relations were taking place it also contributes to our understanding of how to think about *community participation* in rebuilding post-conflict societies. Furthermore, it points out some flaws in the idea of community participation, which has become a buzz word in international development over the last two decades. People's experiences agree with Chernoff's view that "while we are thinking about their [people in this narrative] lives, they are dealing with them" (2003: 8). This provides a cautionary narrative for an international policy discussion which tends to consider target groups as victims, with these victims often framed as passive recipients waiting for international interventions to deal with their problems. The extracts above show that people are anything but passive in engaging with their lives and problems within those lives. The timeline which has emerged above also shows that some of the community groups emerged at the end of 1990s and early 2000s when the conflict was impacting lives and they were observing the way HIV was impacting their communities. In other words, far from being passive they were responding to the dynamically changing needs they had in their own communities. It was not easy. They required action to come together in the midst of a conflict and tackle issues, including HIV. The idea of passive victims waiting to be helped by outsiders was not a reference point in these reflections.

In line with the focus on participation and civil society within the international development fora in the last two decades, many international HIV/AIDS policy debates have focused on participation as an important process, and civil society as one of the central actors for HIV/AIDS interventions (Seckinelgin 2002, 2006, 2008; Duffield 2007: 91). Linked to this overall policy framing, community participation is seen as a way of achieving appropriate framing for interventions, for their sustainability over time, for building ownership for many of these interventions and as a way of sensitization to deal with stigma (Hadley and Maher 2001; Segall 2003; van Wyk *et al.* 2006; Poku and Sandkjaer 2007). These academic discussions are undoubtedly important and they are also attempts to bring communities to deal with their own problems. However, there is an uncomfortable relationship between the international policy context within which these ideas gained currency and people's everyday contexts.

As the extracts above show, people are already actively taking part in their everyday lives both to change their lives and to influence others. In other words they are already participating. Therefore, the participation discussion, as it has emerged within the international policy fora, becomes a problem as the implication is that people should participate in and according to the international HIV/AIDS or in the international DDR policy frameworks. This position ignores the ongoing work that is done on a daily basis by people in their communities. It also assumes a close fit between international policy frameworks and "contextual constraints and possibilities shaping the behavior of target group members" (Campbell and Cornish 2010: 1570). The former assumption creates or feeds the general tendency to assume that communities "lack resources for mobilization" (Campbell and Cornish 2010: 1574). The latter then leads to the facile interventions to build community or civil society groups to facilitate people's participation in international policy schemes.

Another issue emerges at the intersection of these dynamics. International HIV/AIDS policy frameworks target particular groups. Policy incentives for people to participate and create community groups frame the nature of community groups in line with the interests of the policy actors. In other words, these interventions often create community groups in ways that can be identifiably linked with the policy priorities. As a result, the idea of community in these community groups and in their activities is about the way people are differentiated from others according to the policy targeting them. There is no doubt that groups of HIV+ people, groups of ex-combatants, or groups of mothers have relevance in the way these groups have access to services. This kind of belonging allows them to have access to resources provided by formal systems. It is not clear, however, when these groups are taken to represent community activity in this limited sense and how this process abstracts them from belonging to the everyday communities within which they function by relying on socio-cultural resources to maintain their lives. The transposition of communities of policy in the place of communities of everyday life presents important challenges for HIV/AIDS interventions, since it confuses aspects of the community mobilization that are important for people to deal with HIV/AIDS interventions with aspects of community organizations that are relevant for policy makers.

Policy interests slice people's lives up according to their particular interests. As a result one person becomes an object of attention from multiple policy angles without any one of these angles having an overall understanding of their lives. People do not consider their lives in these terms. The reflections presented in this chapter and in the book in general show that people consider their lives as a whole and deal with many problems they face from that position. The example of the ex-combatants' DDR experiences relates to this problem. Once put in the community of ex-combatants and targeted by various services in the demobilization camps individuals are simply expected to integrate. It is not clear, however, why international policy makers assume that people targeted only as fighters in the DDR process will then become or transformed into civilians relating to diverse aspects in their everyday lives.

Lives are always changing. People's lives are part of an overall dynamic and people also act to change their communities' experience. Their active participation in these processes, as demonstrated above, is underlined by a holistic view on life. While community groups, organizations, and their participation have become a mantra, what seems to matter, looking at the extracts, is not the policy label attached to these groups, but rather what people are able to do to influence social change given the socio-cultural contexts they live in.

In a discussion with the director of a local NGO working on human rights-related issues in Bujumbura, she pointed out that to deal with marginalized groups it was important to gain the trust of the larger community through the organization's work before trying to challenge the community's prejudices. Her particular starting point was dealing with street children in urban space. Having done this she explained that they are able to do some work on Twa, the smallest of the three ethnic groups in Burundi and traditionally they are excluded by both Tutsi and Hutu. People refuse to eat in the same place or drink from the same cup as Twa. Her point was that in order to overcome the prejudice one needs to create a social process through which people can come together and develop experiences together so that they can think about a group beyond the basis of an existing prejudice. This is, of course, a long process, and for that reason alone it might not fit with the logic of international aid or policies with their short funding cycles.

To conclude, this chapter has highlighted the mismatch between the way people in communities deal with their everyday problems and the understanding of community work, and organizations within the international policy fora. The research material provided here raises questions for international policy makers and the way they engage with people's experiences. The interview material highlights the kinds of socio-cultural mechanisms utilized and developed through people's community work to influence social change. These experiences identify a cleavage between the way people tried to deal with HIV/AIDS in their communities as a part of their overall well-being needs in the middle of the conflict and also the absence of such engagements in the social context ex-combatants. This cleavage and its implications for ex-combatants' reintegration should inform the DDR process. There is also an absence of this kind of grounded knowledge of people's experiences of community work to inform what matters for sustainable HIV/AIDS-related interventions within international policy thinking. This absence allows policy makers to articulate abstract and top-down characteristics for ideal communities and community action. However, aspirational approaches to help communities evident in the international policy context are likely to fall short of achieving their aims unless the lived experiences of people in particular contexts become part of the grounds for policy knowledge.

Conclusion

The book considered the relationships between conflict and HIV/AIDS. This was done by thinking along with people's experiences of conflict and HIV/AIDS in Burundi. Thinking along provides an important critical corrective to the way the relationship between conflict and HIV/AIDS is typically considered under the international security and the HIV/AIDS framework. I see the research material based on people's reflections on their experiences as an invitation to think critically about international policy context and about the basis of the knowledge which in that context locates people as target groups within an international policy framework (Stone-Mediatore 1998: 129). As I outlined in the introduction, the international security and HIV/AIDS framework has developed into one of the main policy frameworks for engaging with HIV/AIDS since 2000. The book began with the experiences of people rather than beginning with the assumptions that have dominated the international security and HIV/AIDS debate. This reflects that in the context of Burundi I consider people's experiences and reflections on conflict and HIV/AIDS as the main source of knowledge for assessing the socio-cultural mechanisms that mediate conflict processes and vulnerability to HIV. This is done without pre-judging to support either the link between security and HIV/AIDS or not.

The book also raised questions about the way security and HIV/AIDS debate is framed, about how this framing informs the policy implementation and how both of these have failed to address people's needs and wellbeing in the case of Burundi. The book shows that the top-down policy discussions miss the point about the way people experience the disease both during and after the conflict. One of the reasons for this problem is the way both the security and HIV/AIDS discourse and the actual policy implementations approach the issue without paying specific attention to gender relations and people's gendered experiences. Furthermore, the book argues that the attempt to link conflict and HIV through abstract assumptions, developed in international security debates and policies, orients the research to consider superficially observable relations or their absence as discussed in Chapters 6 and 7. These ultimately produce the kind of knowledge which is distanced from the people's everyday experiences without paying attention to their reflections of these experiences as the possible grounds for thinking about policies. Furthermore, any attempt to engage with people is likely to be ineffective without addressing the cognitive world of those targeted.

This book's subtitle, *HIV/AIDS is another war*, captures this kind of located knowledge. The subtitle reflects the way people experience processes of war, how it came about and influenced lives, and the way people think about HIV in an analogous manner. It came out in an interview with a woman who was in her late 40s in a rural commune. She used the phrase in her reflections of how she found out about her HIV status. She said that although she had never left her home, had worked hard in the fields and only had one husband, she had HIV. She said it was like the war, she did not know how it had arrived. But it arrived nonetheless. She also realized that it arrived via her husband who used to travel to sell what they farmed. The analogy with war highlights the complexity of living in the context of HIV in a similar way to living in the context of war. She was pointing out that she was impacted even if she did not know the causes of change. The unexpectedness of both HIV and war for many lives was important. However, the phrase is not intended to express helplessness. It is more about considering these two issues as part of people's lives: to issues in which things unexpectedly happen and people develop ways of dealing with them. She was reflecting on how she assessed her situation in a relational manner. Underlying the assessment are intersections of gender, legal entitlements, financial ability, disease and war framing her life experiences. Her reflections were informed by such a rich view on her life as a whole than simply being a target, as a HIV+ person or as someone who needs to be secured against others. Similar views were also expressed in a group discussion with HIV+ women, presented in Chapter 8. In their reflections there is also a clear sense of unexpectedness about HIV+. However, once they knew their status they tried to influence their communities. They were trying to find ways of talking about it. The subtitle is not intended to suggest there is an uncomplicated direct link between war and HIV in the way it is captured in the security and HIV/AIDS framework. Rather, it captures the way people's lives intersect with each other through everyday lives and how these intersections create conflicts as well as ways to deal with these conflicts. In a way people's reflections are not about security, they recognize the idea of security as fleeting. People are interested in influencing social change and they negotiate conflictual interests as an inevitable part of everyday life.

Contribution of the book: disruptions and methodology

The research material presented in this book disrupts the knowledge claims of the international security experts on HIV/AIDS. It does this by demonstrating a major gap between their articulation of the relationship between conflict and HIV/AIDS and people's experiences of the disease and conflict in Burundi. It further disrupts the way expert knowledge is produced by relying on epistemologically questionable assumptions on people's lives and how these intersect with HIV/AIDS. The mechanism for this disruption is considering a different kind of knowledge that clearly is relevant for thinking about HIV/AIDS and HIV/AIDS in conflict. Doing this lead one to ask what needs to be known understand HIV/AIDS in conflict. This question is in turn linked with the general question of what is required for HIV/AIDS knowledge. The argument in this book also highlights the importance of gender analysis for HIV/AIDS and the importance of this kind of analysis for understanding people's lives in conflict contexts. The HIV virus does not spread by itself, its spread is the function of sexual relations which are a sub-set of broader social relations in a given socio-cultural context. People's reflections provide some of the grounds on which one can understand the social conditions of HIV spread. Therefore, the questions of whose knowledge we are looking at and what we need to consider become important considerations (Code 1994: 13). In other words, if we are interested in HIV and people's experience research needs to begin with questions that are relevant to people's HIV concerns. These considerations attend to the difference between knowledge captured within the international policy frameworks and knowledge that is embedded within people's everyday contexts. This relevance point of view shows HIV/AIDS knowledge is contingent on people's social contexts. If one takes this position seriously it has important implications for the ongoing international policy framing in so far as the international framing discounts people's local knowledge when answering questions that are relevant to international fora (Longino 2010: 734). The methodological move argued for here is best captured by Helen Longino when she argues that:

> the subject of knowledge is no longer ideally disembodied and universal, at least qua knower, but embodied and specific, particular, complex and multiple. This subject of knowledge is located, has perspectives, is shaped by its physical and social locations.
>
> (2010: 736)

The relationship between expert knowledge on HIV/AIDS and the knowledge warranted by living with the disease in a given context becomes a pressing issue international policy makers cannot ignore.

This represents a cleavage between traditional epistemology and a feminist epistemology. The essence of difference is between allowing localized experience to warrant knowledge claims versus the traditional position that is related with rules of inference related to the way the latter declares according to Laura Ruetsche "social contingencies irrelevant to warrant, and so irrelevant to epistemology, the traditionalist assumes that contingencies cannot enter into the constitution of evidential relations" (Ruetsche 2004: 79). According to Ruetsche, the traditional position makes the approach "invariant under changes in social (or historical or natural or …) context. Offering this invariance as at least the mark if not the essence of objectivity" (2004: 77). Given this a proponent of the traditional approach might question the relevance of personal experiences of conflict or HIV as they might be seen as contingent on personal circumstances or emotions about particular experiences. Thus, they are not sufficiently objective or they do not offer sufficiently invariant conditions to consider experiences. However, I would dispute this. I agree with Elizabeth Anderson that emotions are not empty place holders. They relate to "events, things, to states", they represent personal evaluations that are "positive or negative" in relation to these, in these evaluations they indicate a "perspective or point of view of subjects who care about themselves or others" and these "signal the importance of things" that people care about (2004: 9). Paying attention to these in people's reflections on their lives, it is possible to question the grounds on which the hypothesis on the relationship between security and HIV/AIDS is articulated, for example, in the Spiegel *et al.* piece discussed in Chapter 6. The discussions in Chapters 6 and 7 reveal that this hypothesis relies on assumptions that are significantly distanced from what matters to people in their experiences during particular conflicts and their relation to HIV/AIDS in these contexts. The hypothesis is based on the limited context of the international security concerns both at the policy and scholarly levels (Reutsche 2004: 86). Therefore, international policy actors can neither understand nor observe what matters to people in their lives in relation to HIV and conflict.

This conventional approach might be defended by arguments for parsimony at the international level, whereas the approach proposed here might be seen as leading to competing claims and a confusion between truth and emotional reflections. These in turn could be seen as unhelpful for international policy concerns that are trying to intervene in multiple contexts. Again I would disagree. As Longino argues, "tolerance of inconsistent descriptions flowing from differently situated perspectives on a phenomenon enables us to obtain a fuller, more comprehensive understanding than we could from any single one" (2010: 738). Inconsistency is a function of the way people engage with their environment and with changing circumstances. Expectation of consistent approach itself negates differences for the benefit of abstract clarity, in the present case, across different categories of conflicts and different experiences of the disease. Yet people's needs have to be understood within their specific circumstances. Parallel to Reutsche's (2004: 86) consideration of " feminist epistemology" the methodological aim of the book then is to point out that people's experiences in particular socio-cultural contexts influenced by gender relations warrant knowledge claims that are most relevant to think about conflict and HIV/AIDS.

The intersections between conflict processes and people's everyday lives observed in Burundi provide a complex set of pathways to consider implications of conflicts for risk to HIV. People's reflections on their lives were explicitly or implicitly referring to the multi-layered implications of the gender governance in the country before and during the conflict. This position might be questioned by the international policy thinking. One could counter that Burundi represents just one case and as such questions why it should be relevant for international policy concerns on conflict and HIV/AIDS in general. However, this book is not trying to extrapolate substantive knowledge claims about conflicts or HIV/AIDS in general. Instead it highlights how conflict and HIV/AIDS are linked with each other in the case of Burundi. In doing this it also identifies gender relations as a central structural mechanism. It argues that structural mechanisms such as gender are central to any understanding of the vulnerability to and the experiences of HIV/AIDS. This approach does not try to attribute substantive content to these mechanisms in general on the basis of Burundian experience. It provides a way of methodologically thinking about conflict and people's HIV related needs in such contexts. This way of thinking is interested first in people's lives and their experiences of the disease. It then considers the way these lives interact with conflict. The book claims that looking at the questions from this angle reveals the kind of social relations that are important for vulnerability to HIV; and identifies gender governance as a central mechanism for people's sexual behavior that is relevant for vulnerability to HIV. While gender governance is considered to be a vital component for the analysis of HIV/AIDS and people's conflict related behavior, the substantive content of the gender governance determined by norms and values in a given society have to be understood and considered case by case. In other words, the way gender governance regulates social relations and the way this regulation produces particular behavior will vary in each case. Furthermore, the discussion on Burundi cannot be understood independently of the way international policy discussions construct the nature of the conflict in Burundi within their policy narratives, and doing so frame people's HIV/AIDS-related needs. The latter framing is based on the assumed relations between subjectivities as perceived from within the international policy fora. The book's methodological orientation challenges the grounds on which policy makers claim to know about people's behavior in relation to HIV/AIDS and policy thinking in relation to conflict, HIV/AIDS and security. The book provides what Code calls a "healthy skepticism" as a "response to excessive and irresponsible global pretensions, whose excesses have to be communally debated and negotiated with due regard to local specificities and global implications" (1998: 75).

The book conceptually argues that if the vulnerability to HIV is the main concern the lack of gender analysis leads to the simplification of social relations that are relevant for thinking about the conflict and HIV relationship. This lack is a function of the security discourse in general and the way gender is incorporated into security studies. I look at these in turn in the following sections.

Gender-based analysis and HIV/AIDS

As I argued in the introduction, policy thinking on AIDS and security has developed into one of the main international policy frameworks. The knowledge base on which this policy area relies treats it as a sub-set of international security discourse. This is an inappropriate ground to think about people's vulnerability to HIV/AIDS. One of the central reasons for this is that international security discourse has traditionally ignored gender perspectives. As shown in the Burundian case, gender analysis is central to understanding the socio-cultural context of the behavior that is relevant for HIV. It is also central to understand how people are able to engage with the disease and causes of its spread. Most of the gender-based discussions on security emerged as alternatives to the mainstream approaches to security questions. For instance, Laura Sjoberg writing in 2009 observes that "no gender-based article has appeared on the pages of *Security Studies* as of the time [we] are compiling this issue [special issue on feminist contributions]" (2009: 185). This is just one indication of the situation. More importantly, the lack of interest in gender and gender-based analysis is a major handicap to make sense of HIV/AIDS.

The mainstream international security approaches and feminist scholarship have an uneasy relationship. Despite its marginalization, a strong scholarship on gender/feminism and security has developed. The mainstream that is occupied itself with state security interests has reluctantly incorporated some of the views from these alternative positions. Most of this feminist literature has focused on bringing women's experiences into the discussions of security. These moves highlight the previous and largely ongoing lack of concern for women and their experiences within security discussions. Many feminist scholars have looked at case studies to understand how women were impacted by the military and the ways through which soldiers engage with civilians. An important policy landmark here is the United Nations Security Council Resolution 1325 that was adopted in October 2000. This resolution brought feminist concerns about women's experiences in conflict contexts into the heart of the international policy fora. While this move undoubtedly signified a success for many feminist scholars and activists working on security, it also signified a moment at which the feminist discussion and gender-based analysis became part of the conventional security establishment. In a way it shows a pathway through which critique becomes institutionalized as a part of the conventional thinking (Seckinelgin 2008). Given the security mandate of the Security Council, the resolution linked its approach to women directly in relation to peacekeeping operations and personnel taking part in these operations with a special emphasis on how they engage with people by paying attention to women's specialized needs. HIV/AIDS was also incorporated into the security agenda through this mechanism, with the UN Security Council Resolution 1308 in 2000. Here the Security Council expressed its commitment to HIV/AIDS with a new resolution –1983 – on 7 June 2011.

Both gender, mostly women in this case, and HIV/AIDS are firmly securitized (Buzan *et al.* 1997). They are, in other words, a concern for policy makers as regards to international security. These concerns manifest themselves in influencing the kinds of groups that matter for policy actors from an international security perspective. There are a number of variations in this area. For instance, some try to improve the interventions in conflict contexts by introducing women as a new category of relevant group so that their needs are addressed in conflict and post conflict-contexts (Higate and Henry 2004). Another approach is to introduce gender-based analysis to reconstruct new security thinking within the international fora (Alison 2004; Handrahan 2004). In these approaches women and their gendered needs are an addition to the sub-stantively unchanged security policy content. In a similar vein, HIV is mostly considered from the position of peacekeeping or security sector reforms to shape new armies after the conflict and to maintain and balance the security interest of a country and its international position. In this process of the securitization of women's needs and HIV/AIDS men's experiences in conflict are also homogenized. They are concern for policy makers situated within these over-arching policy frameworks so long as men can be considered as soldiers, as members of other armed groups or as guerrillas. The differentiated experi-ences of men and the gendered implications of these on HIV/AIDS are not considered.

Furthermore, there is a tension between acknowledging differentiated experiences of women and using women as a universal category to engage with international policy frameworks (Alexander and Mohanty 1997; see Code 1998: 75). The latter leads to broad brush policy prescriptions based on generic categorical target groups, such as women who are exposed to gender-based violence, orphans and the displaced, those who are prioritized by the international policy. And although some policies focus on women's experi-ences within the limited context of a conflict they do not pay much attention to the overall interactions between socio-cultural contexts and the conflict, which create the context, for instance, rape or displacement. In addition, many of these approaches are not sensitive to intra-woman differences and the varied experiences within given socio-cultural contexts. And while they iden-tify women-specific security needs, these tend to be at the level of broad pat-terns that are open to generalizations for international policy targeting. Problems are presented as representations of all women's experiences in con-flict. They do not provide insights as to the structural conditions that produce and reproduce what they identify as women's security needs. While they emphasize these security needs, the social mechanisms creating these needs through time are omitted from the discussion as policy interventions focus on mitigating the symptoms rather than looking at the underlying causes of these symptoms. Partially, this is due to the way that feminist interventions and gender-based analysis have been trying to engage the meta-theoretical under-standing of security underwriting the international security policies. Research in particular cases is used to extrapolate generic statements of the problems of groups that are targeted by the international policy makers. The motivation to have an impact within the international policy fora leads to abstraction from people's experiences and to inappropriate generalization about people in other conflict contexts. Lena Hansen and Louise Olsson in their introduction to the special issue on Gender and Security for *Security Dialogue* describe the aims of feminist security analysis in two ways: "to critique the field of security studies for its inherent male biases and to trace how particular political practices produce collective conceptualizations that constrict or enable what can be recognized as legitimate problems of the individual" (2004: 405). They also emphasize that their approach considers security as a combination of and as a relationship between individual and collective security concerns. Their approach provides a theoretical move towards linking feminist concerns on women's experiences with gender concerns about the way women's social roles are constructed to inform these experiences. This is a useful way to think in relation to HIV/AIDS as analytically it brings together both the individual and the conditions under which that individual is able to act. This could allow engagement with people's experiences in particular contexts. However, their next move diminishes this potential in their thinking.

They argue that their position is not a "gendered analysis [that] advocates an abandonment of the traditional conception of "military-state security" of realism and strategic studies but rather that it critically studies the production and consequences of this approach" (2004: 406). They then list a set of questions that are relevant for their concerns. An interesting aspect of these questions is that they appear informed mostly by meta-security concerns framed at the national or international level. While they are significantly arguing that "feminist security is transforming questions of military and state security" and it is prioritizing gender over "women's security', they still seem to focus on explaining security and how it is gendered (2004: 406). From a HIV/AIDS perspective, this leads to an analysis which links individual experience in contexts by considering these as relevant within the larger security discussion on, for instance, peacekeeping, foreign troops, and displacement. As relevant as these are, concerns based on these objectify women's particular experiences.

This general approach creates a tension between remaining within the meta-security debates and bringing in a gender-analysis into inform this debate. In this engagement the gender-analysis is incorporated to the discussion to answer questions determined by or referenced to the international security discourse, as can, for instance, be seen within the Security Council's mandate. As a result, the gender-analysis remains attached to the security questions or to an agenda defined independent of people's experiences. The idea of security seems to remain constant in many of these discussions. While these are important interventions, the attachment to the idea of security does not allow a "moving beyond the knowledge frameworks that construct" international security (Tickner 1997: 621). Therefore, the central contributions of feminist epistemologies, as identified by Shumalit Reinharz as "making the invisible visible, bringing women's lives to the center, rendering the trivial important … and understanding women as subjects rather than object of men" are negated (1992: 248). The focus on security as a starting point means that the concerns about security are determined in a top-down manner. As a result, there remains a gap between the abstract gender concerns brought into the international security discussion and the way people unpack their problems and the way these are negotiated/renegotiated in their own socio-cultural contexts. Here the problem is not strictly speaking with feminist/gender research but rather with the way this research is linked to and limited within international security thinking and related policy concerns.

This could be read as a criticism of theory. There is no doubt theoretical knowledge is important in relation to gender concerns and that many gender-theoretic positions provide important challenges to the international security debate. However, it is also important that theorization be grounded within people's experiences and that it reflects what these grounded experiences articulate. There are two central reasons for this: (a) without it there is nothing methodologically to stop gender-based analysis from being incorporated into universalistic approaches that ignore particular experiences; (b) experiences of people that are supposed to be benefitting from these discussions should be the grounds to begin thinking about the problems and issues. Otherwise the instinct to help others is to provide frameworks with global reach targeting the poor, the vulnerable, marginalized and other people who are considered to be in need of external help. This leads to people's disempowerment in their own lives. Even in some cases people's experiences are instrumentalized for international policy interests. Hannah Arendt in her discussion of colonial expansion discusses the nature of the colonial bureaucrat whose instinct to help is tempered by his understanding of what needs people have: "the administrator who ruled by reports and decrees in more hostile secrecy than any oriental despot grew out of a tradition of military discipline in the midst of ruthless and lawless men; for a long time he had lived by the honest, earnest boyhood ideals of a modern knight in shining armor sent to protect helpless and primitive people" (1973: 185–186). While here the administrator is evidently male and a product of a particular patriarchal outlook, unless close attention is given to the way gender-based analysis is incorporated within security debate and the limits of this incorporation, the aspiration of helping others implicit in the normative feminist position can all too easily become a justification for new knights in shining armors (see Duffield 2007: 32–65). In this instinct people's embedded agency is negated and with that their reflections on their lives are also lost as a way of knowing.

Security is a negative concept

This book contributes to the discussions on gender and conflict. I have unpacked the way the international security discourse has framed the HIV/AIDS debate without paying attention to people's experiences. I also draw attention to the relationship between security as a master narrative and gender-based analysis as a critical approach within this meta-narrative. I have argued that the former negates the impact of gender-based analysis, since most discussions on gender and security begin from a limiting normative position when considering the implications of security discourse, or the actual security in a given conflict for women. The innovation presented in these approaches tends to be about ways of thinking on how to address women's security needs. As important as these are, they tend to assert a certain coherence about the nature of being women in insecure environments. They rarely unpack the actual mechanisms creating the insecurity in particular the socio-cultural contexts. Furthermore, they do not engage with the implications of considering the particularized needs of people from a security perspective. This book, in contrast, argues that looking at security from a gender perspective needs to question the security discussion and its foundation. Here the claim is not about the actual instances of insecurity that are considered in relation to particular violent episodes. Rather the argument is about the way the logic of security is applied a-temporally and broadly to intervene on behalf of people, groups or individuals. I now discuss this further.

Security is a negative and a relational concept. Put simply, it aims to secure a thing, a group or individuals against something else or some others. The aim is to create conditions for survival independent of, or against, those people (or things) who are identified as the possible causes disrupting such survival. With this basis it is possible to consider security in all the walks of life that are linked with survival needs. In its more conventional form the possibility of providing security to a group is also seen as a legitimating factor for claiming political authority. Moreover the possibility of enforcing security within that group to secure individuals against each other and enforcing it externally to defend that group's security are also seen as the condition for political authority. While this suggests that security is a temporal concept, the ability to secure has become a permanent quality for political legitimacy and the question of responsibility within the international arena. In most of these discussions the target groups that require securing are determined by the authority that claims to have the ability to secure. Therefore security is not only a negative concept that is always about mutually exclusive states of being, but also a disempowering concept. It legitimates the authority of the actors claiming to have the capacity to secure at the expense of the agency of those secured.

This is often done under the claims of supporting groups" or people's survival. Those who are secured are seen as giving their tacit consent for this state of affairs. However, it is often unclear what people think about their situation and the way they are secured. In other words, people's lives are reframed from the position of the actor who is doing the securing. As Maria Stern argues, "securing the subject requires 'policing of boundaries' and the 'taming' or homogenisation of an imagined 'self'"(2006: 193). The securitisation process allows these mechanisms to be utilized by declaring subjects that are targeted to be in a state of existential danger unless they are secured (Buzan *et al.* 1997). This means that a group that is secured is cordoned off from others, "contained, nameable, with contours dividing the included from the excluded" (Stern 2006: 192; also see Fassin and Pandolfi 2010). Jeff Huysmans (1995) argues that an issue becomes a concern for security thinking and apparatus, normal politics is suspended, and the politics of exception regulates the circumstances. This also creates a question on the temporality of such claims of danger (see Makaremi 2010; McFalls 2010). At which point does this danger disappear and who decides when the circumstances have changed. The nature of the perceived threat is conceptualized as an existential state, allowing these processes to be considered less critically over time. In this way, the idea of security turns into a permanent state of engaging with particular issues.

This is particularly questionable in relation to the way HIV/AIDS is said to be securitized. Singling groups of people out as security risk for the rest of the society (Elbe 2009; 138–149) ignores the way people engage with unexpected events in their lives. The disease is experienced as a part of overall life course in communities. People with the disease face many problems including stigma. There is no doubt that stigma represents a conflictual relationship between different people or groups of people. People engage and negotiate in their communities when dealing with their problems through the different social spaces open to them, not only as people with HIV but also as members of the community in other ways. Social change in general is the result of negotiation processes within communities over time as responses to events in the life of communities. The securitization of various policy areas such as HIV/AIDS intervenes in these processes. Yet, it does not provide an alternative, a coherent way of dealing with problems in a given context. Instead the international policy based on securitization establishes people with HIV as a distinct group thereby implicitly suggesting that they represent a risk to the community. This kind of policy stalls the existing communication channels within communities by focusing on people, purely on the basis of their HIV status. It reduces the complex linkages underwriting people's belonging in a community to one aspect of their lives. Therefore, policies lead to fragmentation rather than cohesion in communities. They do not support, or build on, the existing spaces and pathways to negotiate and resolve, for instance, the disease-based conflicts in a given society. Arguably, as they distribute resources only to their target groups in this case people with HIV or ex-combatants, they exacerbate tensions in communities.

Some might argue that I should be talking about human security rather than traditional security (Roberts 2006; Sørenson 2007; Glaisus 2008; Chandler 2008a; Ambrosetti 2008; Owen 2008; Wibben 2008). They would point out that my methodological worries and gender orientation lead to issues on people's socio-economic needs. These moves to "re-evaluate traditional security politics are not covered by conventional security politics … a reorientation of security dynamic … moves the concept of security away from patriarchal and hierarchal structure in which the prevailing security discourse is encased" and that this would allow one "to recognise ways in which these securities are linked to one another, rather than isolating them from one another and prioritising them individually" (Hoogensen and Rottem 2004: 167–168; Fox 2004). Gunhild Hoogensen and Kirsti Stuvøy, for instance, insist that "security must begin with the individual" and then argue for a redefinition of security as in Basch, "freeing individuals and groups from social, physical, economic and political constraints that prevent them from carrying out what they would freely choose to do" (2004: 21; Basch 2004: 9). Colleen O'Manique (2005) indeed considers securitization of HIV/AIDS from a human security perspective. She argues that the current securitisation of the disease ignores the "the broader contributions to human insecurity located in current global distribution of power and resources" (2005: 26). She then points out how human security concept emerged from feminist studies of traditional security. She defines human security as "the absence of violence, whether sexual, military, environmental or economic; whether it originates from relationships within the household, from economic restructuring, from the national security policies of particular states (2005: 26). Her approach then used to engage with "security crisis of AIDS" (2005: 26). In this feminist approach the local, "everyday lived experiences" and the experiences of power at multiple levels are relevant grounds for analysis.

There is no doubt that the human security discussion has brought many other concerns about human condition to the security debate challenging the traditional security view. Women and HIV/AIDS, as pointed out before via the UN Security Council, are two important areas considered as being securitized. However, I would argue that this expansion of security agenda does not mean that the logic of security as a negative and disempowering approach has been changed. For instance, the list provided above by Hoogensen and Stuvøy keeps the debate in the logic of security unless there are unlimited resources to allow these resource constraints to be removed for everyone. Otherwise how will one secure their economic or political needs without juxtaposing their interests against some others. Posed as a security issue these concerns become mutually exclusive domains of interests for people.

Similarly in a recent work, Shannon D. Beebe and Mary Kaldor describe their understanding of human security as being "about the everyday security of individuals and the communities in which they live rather than security of states and borders" (2010: 5). They then provide a list of principles which should be used in dealing with security problems (Beebe and Kaldor 2010: 8–9). They seem to take human security as a part of the goal of international interventions and that the principles then considered guaranteeing its delivery for dealing with violence experienced by civilians. This aim is clearly linked with their assumption that the "human security approach aims at preventing an escalation of violence" (Beebe and Kaldor 2010: 89). This shows how the human security approach is different from the traditional security approach in degrees rather than in kind. Although it might be changing the way the security apparatus functions and operates in civilian context, it is not clear how far the negative logic of security is challenged. Indeed, although Beebe and Kaldor are interested in violence against civilians and not the security of states, implicitly it seems that they see human security as a means to achieve and underwrite just such traditional security concerns. The principles of human security that are outlined in their work can be seen as the restatement of traditional security logic with a civilian mandate. These principles are the expansion of security logic to everyday life in relation to livelihoods.

These discussion underwrite the impasse between the interests of international policy actors and the way people engage with their lives. For instance, O'Manique in her conclusion is still trying to provide a "feminist lens" focusing on "AIDS and security crisis" (2005: 43). She is asserting very clearly that "genuine human security is conditional upon the women who continue to struggle for their security, and the security of their families in the context of the exercise of basic human rights" (2005: 43-44). This is a curious ending for an argument which clearly argued for the analysis of local and lived experiences of people. It seems to have already formed a view as to what it means to have human security as a function of particular security threats; there does not seem to be much space here for local and lived experiences to raise questions about this human security framing. While these discussions focus on human interests to counter a generic state interest based discussion of security, a generalized view of humans and the human condition are nonetheless assumed. In other words a generic, an abstract, idea of human with universalized needs, is relied upon. It is not clear, how, for instance, the human security position can engage with the questions on: when people in particular contexts feel secure in their everyday lives. Given the complex livelihood conditions of those living in conflict, from a human security perspective they may never escape the human security zone that is now all encompassing. Their lives become a matter for development interventions as an extension of, and to maintain human security (Duffield 2007). The move towards human security is not a move away from security and its politics. David Chandler argues that "what [I] find most worrying is the attempt to portray the human security policy discourse as somehow marginal to the articulation of power and the frameworks of international regulation and intervention today" (2008b: 465). In short the human security discourse does not seem to recognize its family resemblance to existing discourses in which the interests of people everywhere are framed within a politics of inclusion and exclusion, disempowering local agency to live in different ways.

Living in communities vs. security

This book has identified a major gap between lived experiences and the way international policies are structured, targeting what they identify as problems in people's lives in general. Leaving aside all the conceptual problems attached to the concept of security and human security, it is clear that people's narratives of their experiences of conflict and HIV do not use the kind of security language that is common within the international policy fora. Does this matter? People talk about instances of violence, being hungry or homeless and insecure during the conflict. After the conflict they point out hunger, disease and lack of work as major problems in their lives. They also talk about the criminality created during the conflict and how this is impacting social change in the society which is trying to come to terms with the effects of the conflict (Uvin 2009: 46). These reflections provide a dynamic understanding of their lives in changing circumstances. Peter Uvin talks about these issues in relation to the perceptions of peace in Burundi. In his work it is clear that people's perception of peace is multi-layered and does not just consider peace as an absence of war but as a constant process of building their lives and their communities. He classifies the various ways peace was articulated by people in his research "peace as safety, as basic needs, as social peace, and as good governance" (2009: 43–57). In this classification there is also an implicit ordering. People like to live without criminality and violence that were generated by the conflict, they want to have enough to support their livelihoods, then they consider the importance of "cohabitation, social harmony" (2009: 48). Some of our interviewers also talked about how resources are managed and distributed in the country (in my research as we were interested in HIV/ AIDS resource distribution issues were very much part of many people's reflections). Uvin argues that the classification he produced does not create a composite idea of peace but they rather reflect the differentiated views coming from people's different experiences. He also points out that the superficial resemblance between these highlighted issues and the way the international agenda is focusing on "security, development and restoration of social relations" (2009: 51). He then points out that this resemblance loses its usefulness as a way of thinking once the substance of these views and how people are trying to achieve them are unpacked. He says that "it is one thing to be on the same wavelength regarding the overall direction, and quite another to implement [this] in concrete actions (Uvin 2009: 52).

This point identifies a major problem associated with the way international top-down frameworks in their attempt to consider local conditions reduce contextual reflections, differences and aspirations to reference points they have within their way of thinking. This raises the question of whether it is enough to identify similarities between international interests and what these interests interpret local experiences to be, to go ahead and to develop policies for interventions. People might very well be talking about things which go under a generalized category of basic needs and social peace, but the actual content of these differ from what these categories indicate within the international frameworks. Similarly people's concerns for safety might be taken as an indication of their demand for security. People's concern for safety indicates a kind of security that facilitates their social engagements to negotiate and re-negotiate their social relations. This is different from the way international policy looks at the security and attempts to create zones of exceptions for particular groups. The social relations people talk about serve many functions tied within a living community rather than just being secured against each other.

People's reflections also indicate a much more dynamic engagement with their environment even within the processes of conflict. They recognize the essentially conflictual nature of social relations. As a result, their aspirations are about dealing with conflict to develop a way of living together in communities. Because of this, the view of securing people to maintain their lives falls short of understanding that people's life considerations present coherence of their lives in the broader context of their communities. The divergence here is also clear from the way people's reflections demonstrate that people have agency and they influence social change. Even in the midst of violence, for instance, women's reflection about IDP camps and their conditions articulate the ways they assessed what mattered to them and how they navigated the constraints created by these settlements. Furthermore, many women's reluctance to go through the DDR process were based on similar calculations. In the same vein people's engagement with HIV/AIDS, as discussed in the last chapter but also clear in others, indicate that people are "active" and they make "urgent attempts to solve problems they face" (Cotts *et al.* 2009: 173). These show on the one hand women's agency and the evaluations they arrive at about the circumstances at certain moments in time. They reflect that these evaluations were their assessment of life choices based on their experiences, including sexual exploitation, and considerations of what the implications of these will be for them in the social continuum they have to exist in. On the other hand they bear witness to the shortsightedness of many international interventions that are constructing people's according to their categorical interests without considering coherence of lives and their intersections within social relations. At the end people want to deal with conflict by finding a common ground within their communities not by securing themselves against each other.

Bibliography

Achebe, N. and Teboh, B. (2007) 'Dialoguing Women' in C. M. Cole, T. Manuh, S. F. Miescher (eds) *Africa After Gender?* Bloomington: Indiana University Press.

African Crisis (AC) (2010) *Burundi: HIV-Positive People Struggling for Treatment – August 11*. www.africancrisis.co.za/Article.php?ID=81158Introduction: Genealogy, Legacies, Movements' in M. J. Alexander and C. T. Mohanty (eds) *Feminist Genealogies, Colonial Legacies, Democratic Futures*. New York: Routledge.

Alison, M. (2004) 'Women as Agents of Political Violence: Gendering Security' *Security Dialogue* Vol. 35, 4: 447–63.

Allen, T. (2006) 'AIDS and evidence: interrogating some Ugandan myths', *Journal of Biosocial* Vol. 38: 7–28.

Altman, D. (2003) 'AIDS and Security', *International Relations* Vol. 17, 3, pp. 417–27.

Altman, D. (2011) Presentation at UNAIDS-IAS meeting on Political science and HIV/AIDS in April 2011 in Bangkok.

Ambrosetti, D. (2008) 'Human Security as Political Resource: A Response to David Chandler's "Human Security: The Dog That Didn't Bark' Security Dialogue Vol. 39, 4: 439–44.

Anderson, E. (2004) 'Uses of Value Judgements in Science: A general Argument, with Lessons from a Case Study of Feminist Research on Divorce,' *Hypatia* Vol. 19, 1: 1–24.

Atran, S. (2010) *Talking to The Enemy: Voice Extremism, Sacred Values and What it Means to be Human*. London: Allen Lane.

Bacchi, C. L. (1999) *Women, Policy and Politics: The Construction of Policy Problems*. London: Sage.

Bacchi, C. (2009) *Analyzing Policy: What's the Problem Presented to Be?* Australia: Pearson Education.

Barnett, A. and Prins, G. (2005) *HIV/AIDS and Security: Fact, Fiction and Evidence* Geneva: UNAIDS.

Basch, L. (2004) 'Human Security, Globalization, and Feminist Visions' *Peace Review* Vol. 16, 1: 5–12.

Beebe, S. D. and Kaldor, M. (2010) *The Ultimate Weapon is no Weapon: Human Security and the New Rules of War and Peace*. New York: Public Affairs.

Bennett, O., Bexley J. and Warnock, K. (1995) *Arms to Fight, Arms to Protect: Women Speak out About Conflict*. London: Panos Publications.

Blanchard, E. M. (2003) 'Gender, International Relations and the Development of Feminist security Theory', *Journal of Women in Culture and Society*, Vol. 28, 4: 1289–1312.

Bratt, D. (2002) Blue Condoms: The Use of International Peacekeepers in the fight against AIDS. *International Peacekeeping*, Vol. 9, 3: 67–86.

Brett, R. (2004) 'Girl Soldiers: Denial of Rights and Responsibilities' *Refugee Survey Quarterly* Vol. 23, 2: 30–37.

Brownson, R. C., Baker, E. A., Leet, T. L., and Gillespie, K. N. (2003) *Evidence-Based Public Health*. Oxford: OUP.

Buzan, B., Wæver, O. and Wilde, J. de (1997) *Security: A New Framework for Analysis*. Boulder, CO: Lynne Rienner Publishers.

Campbell, C. (2003) *Letting Them die: Why HIV Interventions Fail*. Oxford: James Currey.

Campbell, C. and Cornish, F. (2010) 'Towards a "fourth generation" of approaches to HIV/AIDS management: creating contexts for effective community mobilisation' *AIDS Care* Vol. 22, 2: 1569–79.

Campbell, C, Gibbs, A, Maimane, S, Nair, Y., and Sibiya, Z. (2009) Youth participation in the fight against AIDS in South Africa: from policy to practice. *Journal of Youth Studies* Vol. 12, 1: 93–109

Cartwright, N. (2007) *Hunting Causes and Using Them: Approaches in Philosophy and Economics*. Cambridge: Cambridge University Press.

Cartwright, N. (with J. Stegenga) (2008) *A Theory of Evidence for Evidence-Based Policy*. London: the Contingency And Dissent in Science Project Centre for Philosophy of Natural and Social Science, LSE. www.lse.ac.uk/collections/CPNSS/projects/ContingencyDissentInScience/DP/DPCartwright0808TheoryofEvidenceOnline.pdf.

Carver, T. (1996) *Gender Is Not a Synonym for Women*. Boulder, CO: Lynne Rienner.

Chalmers, I. (2005) 'If evidence-informed policy works in practice, does it matter if it doesn't work in theory?' *Evidence & Policy* Vol. 1, 2: 227–42.

Chandler, D. (2008a) 'Human Security: The Dog That Didn't Bark' *Security Dialogue* Vol. 39, 4: 427–38.

——(2008b) 'Human Security II: Waiting for the Tail To Wag the Dog-A rejoinder to Ambrosetti, Owen and Wibben' *Security Dialogue* Vol. 39, 4: 463–69.

Charles, N. and Hintjens, H. M. (1998) *Gender, Ethnicity and Political Ideologies*. New York: Taylor and Francis.

Chernoff, J. (2003) *Hustling is not Stealing: Stories of an African Bar Girl*. Chicago, IL: University of Chicago Press.

Chrétien, J. P. (2002) *The Great Lakes of Africa: Two Thousand Years of History*. New York: Zone Book.

——(2008) 'The Recurrence of Violence in Burundi: Memories of the "Catastrophe" of 1972', in J. P. Chrétien and R. Banegas (eds) *The Recurring Great Lakes Crisis: Identity, Violence and Power*. London: Hurst.

Christie, R. (2010) 'Critical Voices and Human Security: To Endure, To Engage or To Critique?' *Security Dialogue* Vol. 41, 2: 169–90.

CNN (2000), 'U.S. Steps up global fight against AIDS' 10 January, http://archives.cnn.com/2000/US/01/10/aids.africa.02/ (accessed October 2009).

Cockburn, C. 1998. *The Space between Us: Negotiating Gender and National Identities in Conflict*. London: Zed Books.

Code, L. (1994) 'Responsibility and Rhetoric' *Hypatia* Vol. 9, 1: 1–20.

——(1998) 'How to Think Globally: Streching the Limits of Imagination' *Hypatia* Vol. 13, 2: 73–85.

Connell, R. W. (1996) *Masculinities*. London: Polity Press.

Coulter, C., Persson, M., and Utas, M. (2008) *Young Female Fighters in African Wars: Conflict and Its Consequences*. Uppsala: Nordiska Afrikainstitutet.

Daley, P. O. (2008) *Gender & Genocide in Burundi: The Search for Spaces of Peace in the Great Lakes Region*. Oxford: James Currey.

Daston, L. and Galison, P. (2007) *Objectivity*. New York: Zone Books.

De Waal, A., Klot, J. and Mahajan, M. (2009) *HIV/AIDS, Conflict and Security: New Realities, New Responses*. New York: Social Science Research Council.

Dopson, S., Locock, L., Gabbay, J., Ferlie, E., and Fitzgeral, L. (2005) 'Evidence-based Health Care and the Implementation Gap'. In S. Dopson and L. Fitzgerald (eds) *Knowledge to Action? Evidence-Based Health Care in Context*. Oxford: Oxford University Press.

Duffield, M. (2007) *Development, Security and Unending War: Governing the World of Peoples*. Cambridge: Polity Press.

Dyer, C. (2010) *Lancet Retracts MMR paper. BMJ British Medical Journal*. www.bmj.com/cgi/content/full/340/feb02_4/c696.

Elbe, Stefan (2002), 'HIV/AIDS and the Changing Landscape of War in Africa', *International Security* Vol. 27, 2: 159–77.

——(2006) 'Should HIV/AIDS be Securitized? The Ethical Dilemmas of Linking HIV/AIDS and Security', *International Studies Quarterly* 50, 1: 119–44.

——(2009) *Virus Alert: Security, Governmentality and The AIDS Pandemic*. New York: Columbia University Press.

Elshtain, J. B. (1987) *Women and War*. Chicago, IL: The University of Chicago Press.

Enloe, C. (2000) *Maneuvers: The International Politics of Militarizing Women's Lives*. Berkeley: University of California Press.

——(2007) *Globalization and Militarism: Feminist Make the Link*. New York: Rowan and Littlefield.

Falch, Å. (2010) *Women's Political Participation and Influence in Burundi and Nepal*. PRIO Paper (May). Oslo: Peace Research Institute. www.prio.no/sptrans/-80363262 4/Womens-Political-Participation.pdf

Farmer, P. (2009) '"Landmine Boy" and the Tomorrow of Violence', in B. Rylko-Bauer, L. Whiteford and P. Farmer (eds) *Global Health in Times of Violence*. Santa Fe, NM: School for Advanced Research Press.

Fassin, D. (2007) When *Bodies Remember: Experiences and Politics of AIDS in South Africa*. Berkeley: University of California Press.

Fassin D. and Pandolfi M. (eds) (2010) *Contemporary States of emergency: The Politics of Military and Humanitarian Interventions*. New York: Zone Books.

Fox, M.-J. (2004) 'Girls Soldiers: Human Security and Gendered Insecurity' *Security Dialogue* Vol. 35, 4: 465–79.

Frey, W. and Boshoff, H. (2005) 'Burundi's DDR and The Consolidation of Peace'. *African Security Review* Vol. 14. No 4 www.iss.co.za/pubs/ASR/14No4/AWFrey.htm.

Fuest, V. (2008) '"This is Time to Get in Front": Changing Roles and Opportunities for Women in Liberia', *African Affairs* 107, 427: 201–24.

Gibbs, A. (2010) 'Understanding of gender and HIV in the South African media' *AIDS Care* 22, 2: 1620–28.

Glasius, M. (2008) 'Human Security from Paradigm Shift to Operationalization: Job Descriptions for a Human Security Worker' *Security Dialogue* 39, 1: 31–54.

Gregson, S., Adamson, A., Papaya, S., Chimadzwa, T., Mundondo, J., Nyamukapa, C., and Anderson, R. (2007) 'Impact and process evaluation of integrated community and clinic-based HIV1 control: A cluster-randomised trial in eastern Zimbabwe' *PLoS Medicine* 4: 0545–55.

Gruber, J, and Caffrey, M. (2005) 'HIV/AIDS and community conflict in Nigeria: Implications and challenges' *Social Science and Medicine* Vol. 60, 6: 1209–18.

Hadley, M., and Maher, D. (2001) 'Community involvement in tuberculosis control: Lessons from other care programs' *International Journal of Tuberculosis and Lung Disease* 5: 489–90.

Hall, S. (1992) 'The Question of Cultural Identity' in S. Hall, D. Held and A. McGrew (eds) *Modernity and its Futures.* Cambridge: Polity.

Hammersley, M. (1995) *The Politics of Social Research*, London: Sage Publications.

Hammersley, M. (2005) Is the evidence-based practice movement doing more good than harm? Reflections on Iain Chalmers' case for research-based policy making and practice. *Evidence and Policy* 1, 1: 85–100.

Handrahan, L. (2004) 'Conflict, Gender, Ethnicity and Post-Conflict Reconstruction' *Security Dialogue* 35, 4: 429–45.

Hansen, L. (2000) 'The little Mermaid's Silent Security Dilemma and the Absence of Gender in the Copenhagen School', *Millennium-Journal of International Studies* 29: 285–306.

Hansen, L. and Olsson, L. (2004) 'Guest Editors' Introduction' *Security Dialogue* 35, 4: 405–9.

Harriss-White, B. (2005) 'Destitution and the poverty of its Politics-With Special Reference to South Asia', *World Development* 33, 6: 881–91.

Heymann, D. (2003) 'The evolving Infectious Disease Threat: implications for national and global security', *Journal of Human Development* 4, 2: 191–207.

Higate, P. and Henry, M. (2004) 'Engendering (In)security in Peace Support Operations' *Security Dialogue* 35, 4: 481–98.

Hoogensen, G. and Rottem, S. V. (2004) 'Gender Identity and the Subject of Security' *Security Dialogue* 35, 2: 155–71.

Hoogensen, G. and Stuvøy, K. (2006) 'Gender, Resistance and Human Security' *Security Dialogue* 37, 2: 207–28.

Hope, T. (2009) The Illusion of control: A response to Professor Sherma. *Criminology and Criminal Justice* 9 (1): 125–34.

Houlbrook, M. (2005) *Queer London: Perils and Pleasures in the Sexual Metropolis, 1918–1957.* Chicago, IL: The University of Chicago Press.

Hudson, H. (2009) 'Peacebuilding Through a Gender Lens and the Challenges of Implementation in Rwanda and Côte d'Ivoire' *Security Studies* 18, 2: 287–318.

Human Rights Watch (HRW) (2010) *Burundi: Violence, Rights Violations Mar Elections.* July 1. www.hrw.org/en/news/2010/07/01/burundi-violence-rights-violations-mar-elections

Huysmans, J. (1995) 'Migrants as a security Problem: dangers of "Securitizing" Societal Issues' in R. Miles and D. Thranhardt (eds) *Migration and European Integration: Dynamics of Inclusion and Exclusion.* London: Pinter.

Hynes, M. Ward, J., Robertson, K. and Crouse, C. (2004) 'A determination of the Prevalence of Gender-based Violence among conflict-affected populations in east Timor'. *Disasters* 28, 3: 294–321.

International Crisis Group (ICG) (2001) *Burundi: Breaking the Deadlock.* Brussels: International Crisis Group.

IRIN (2007) 'Burundi: HIV/AIDS programmes dealt a severe blow'. www.plusnews. org/report.aspx?ReportId=75835.

——(2008) 'Burundi: HIV programmes suffer as government, NGOs feel the pinch' Bujumbura, 24 October. www.plusnews.org/report.aspx?ReportId=81105

——(2010) 'Burundi: HIV-positive people struggling for treatment of opportunistic infections', Bujumbura, 12 August. www.plusnews.org/Report.aspx?ReportId=90128

Jacobs, S., Jacobson, R., and Marchbank, J. (2000) *States of Conflict: Gender, Violence and Resistance*. London: Zed Books.

Jewkes, R. (2007) 'Comprehensive response to rape needed in conflict settings'. *The Lancet* 369 (9 June): 2140–41.

Kaldor, M. (2007) *Human Security*. Cambridge: Polity Press.

Kandiyoti, D. (1988) Special Issue to Honor Jessie Bernard. *Gender and Society*, 2, 3: 274–290.

Kiefer, L., Frank, J., Di Ruggiero, E., Dobbins, M., Manuel, D., Gully, P. R., and Mowat, D. (2005) 'Fostering Evidence-based decision-making in Canada: Examining the need for a Canadian Population and Public Health Evidence Centre and Research Network'. *Canadian Journal of Public Health* 96, 3: 1–20.

Koss, M. P. (1992) 'The under-detection of rape: methodological choices influence incidence estimates'. *Journal of Social Issues* 48: 61–75

Lemarchand, R. (2009) *The Dynamics of Violence in Central Africa*. Philadelphia, PA: University of Pennsylvania Press.

Lemarchand, R. and David M. (1974) 'Selective Genocide in Burundi,' *Minority Rights Report 20*. London: Minority Rights Group Ltd.

Lindsey, C. (2001) *Women Facing War: ICRC Study on the Impact of Armed Conflict on Women*. ICRC: Geneva.

MacKenzie, M. (2009) 'Securitization and Desecuritization: Female Soldiers and the Reconstruction of Women in Post-conflict Sierra Leone' *Security Studies* Vol. 18, 2, pp. 241–61.

MacLean, S. J., Black, D. R., and Shaw, T. M. (2006) *A Decade of Human Security: Global Governance and New Multilateralism*. London: Ashgate.

Makaremi, C. (2010) 'Utopias of Power: For Human Security to the Responsibility to Protect' in D. Fassin and M. Pandolfi (eds) *Contemporary States of Emergency: The Politics of Military and Humanitarian Interventions*. New York: Zone Books, 107–28.

Mannell, J. (2010). Gender mainstreaming practice: Considerations for HIV/AIDS community organisations. *AIDS Care*, 22(S2), 1613–19.

McFalls, L. (2010) 'Benevolent Dictatorship: The formal Logic of Humanitarian Government' in D. Fassin and M. Pandolfi (eds) *Contemporary States of emergency: The Politics of Military and Humanitarian Interventions*. New York: Zone Books.

McInnes, C. and Rushton, S. (2010) 'HIV, AIDS and security: where are we know?', *International Affairs* 86, 1: 225–45.

McKay and Mazurana (2004) *Where are the girls? Girls in fighting Forces in Northern Uganda, Sierra Leone and Mozambique: Their lives during and after War*. Montreal: Rights and Democracy Institute.

Mertus, J. (2000) *War's Offensive on Women: The Humanitarian Challenge in Bosnia, Kosovo and Afghanistan*. West Hartford: Kumarian Press.

Morgan, M. S. (2008) '"Voice" and the Facts and Observations of Experience' in *Working papers on the Nature of Evidence: How Well Do 'Facts' Travel* No 31/08. LSE.

Moser, C. and Clark, F. C. (2001) *Victims, Perpetrators or Actors? Gender, Armed Conflict and Political*. London: Pakgrave Macmillan.

Mullen, E. J., Shlonsky, A., Bledsoe, E., Bellamy, J. L. (2005) 'From concept to implementation: challenges facing evidence-based social work'. *Evidence and Policy* 1, 1: 61–84.

Multi-Country Demobilization and Reintegration Program (MDRP) (2009) *MDRP Supported Activities in Burundi – December 2008.* www.mdrp.org/PDFs/MDRP_BUR_FS_1208.pdf.

——(2006) *Multi-Country Demobilization and Reintegration Program-Quarterly Progress Report.* www.mdrp.org/PDFs/2006-Q4-QPR-MDRP_XSUM.pdf.

Nnaemeka, O. (1998) *Female Circumcision and The Politics of Knowledge: African women in Imperialist Discourses.* New Jersey: African World Press.

Nordstorm, C. (2009) 'Fault Lines' in B. Rylko-Bauer, L. Whiteford and P. Farmer (eds) *Global Health in Times of Violence.* Santa Fe, NM: School for Advanced Research Press.

Oakley, A., Gough, D., Oliver, S., Thomas, J. (2005) 'lThe politics of evidence and methodology: lessons from the EPPI-Centre'. *Evidence and Policy* 1, 1: 5–31.

O'Manique, C. (2005) 'The "Securitisation of HIV/AIDS in Sub-Saharan Africa: A Critical Feminist Lens', *Policy and Society* 24, 1: 24–47.

Liotta, P. H. (2002) 'Boomerang Effect: The Convergence of national and Human Security', *Security Dialogue* 33, 4: 473–88.

Longino, H. E. (1990) *Science as Social Knowledge: Values and Objectivity in Scientific Inquiry.* Princeton, NJ: Princeton University Press.

——(2010) 'Feminist Epistemology at Hypatia's 25th Annviversary' *Hypatia* 25, 4: 733–41.

MacKinnon, C. A. (2006). *Are Women Human? And Other International Dialogues.* London: Belknap Press of Harvard University Press.

Ostergard, R. L. (2002) 'Politics in the hot zone: AIDS and national security in Africa', *Third World Quarterly* 23, 2: 333–50.

Owen, T. (2008) 'The Critique That Doesn't Bite: a Response to David Chandler's "Human Security: the Dog That Didn't Bark"' *Security Dialogue* 39, 4: 445–53.

Pankhurst, D. (2008) 'Introduction: Gendered War and Peace', in Donna Pankhurst (ed.) *Gendered Peace.* London: Routledge.

Parkhurst, J. O. (2008) '"What worked?": The Evidence Challenges in Determining the Causes of HIV Prevalence Decline' *AIDS Education and Prevention* 20, 3: 275–83.

Peterson, S. (2002) 'Epidemic disease and National Security', *Security Studies* 12, 3: 43–81.

Petticrew, M. and Roberts, M. (2007) Evidence, hierarchies, and typologies: horses for courses. *Journal of Epidemiology and Community Health* 57: 527–29.

Pézard, S. and Florquin, N. (2007) *Small Arms in Burundi: Disarming the Civilian Population in Peacetime. Geneva: the Small Arms Survey* www.smallarmssurvey.org/fileadmin/docs/C-Special-reports/SAS-SR07-Burundi-EN.pdf

Pistorius, P., Gergen, G., and Willershausen, B. (2003) 'Survey about the knowledge of the HIV infection amongst recruits of the German military', *European Journal of Medical Research* 8, 4: 154–60.

Poku, N. and Sandkjaer, B. (2007) 'Meeting the challenges of scaling up HIV/AIDS treatment in Africa' *Development in Practice* 17: 279–90.

Puechguirbal, N. (2010) 'Discourses on Gender, Patriarchy and Resolution 1325: A Textual Analysis of UN Documents', *International Peacekeeping* 17, 2: 172–187.

Rehn, E. and Johnson-Sirleaf, E. (2002)*Women, War and Peace: The Independent Experts' Assessment on the Impact of Armed Conflict on Women and Women's role in Peace-building.* New York: UNDP.

Reyntjens, F. (2006) 'Briefing: Burundi: A Peaceful Transition after a Decade of War', *African Affairs* 105, 418: 117–35.

Roberts, D. (2006) 'Human Security or Human Insecurity? Moving the Debate Forward' *Security Dialogue* 37, 2: 249–61.

Rowley, E. A., Spiegel, P. B., Tunze Z., Mbaruku G., Schilperoord, M., and Njogu P. (2008) Differences in HIV-related behaviors at Lugufu refugee camp and surrounding host villages, Tanzania. *Conflict and Health* Vol. 3:13.

Ruetsche, L. (2004) 'Virtue and Contingent History: Possibilities for Feminist Epistemology' *Hypatia* 19, 1: 73–101.

Seckinelgin, H. (2002) 'Time to Stop and Think: HIV/AIDS, Global Civil Society, and People's Politics' in H. Anheier, M. Glasius and M. Kaldor (eds) *Global Civil Society Year Book 2002*. Oxford: Oxford University Press.

——(2006) 'The Multiple Worlds of NGOs and HIV? AIDS: Rethinking NGOs and Their Agency' *Journal of International Development* Vol. 18.

——(2007) 'Evidence-based Policy for HIV/AIDS Interventions: Questions of External Validity, or Relevance for use' *Development and Change* 38, 6: 1219–34.

——(2008) *International Politics of HIV/AIDS: Global Disease-Local Pain*. London: Routledge.

Seckinelgin, H., Bigirumwami, J., and Morris, J. (2010) 'Securitization of HIV/AIDS in context: gendered vulnerability in Burundi'. *Security Dialogue* 41, 5: 515–35.

Segall, M. (2003) 'District health systems in a neoliberal world: A review of five key areas' *International Journal of Health Planning Management* 18: S5–S26.

Sherman, L. L. (2009) Evidence and liberty: The Promise of Experimental Criminology. *Criminology and Criminal Justice* 9, 1: 5–28.

Singer, P. W. (2002) 'AIDS and International Security', *Survival* 44, 1: 145–58.

Sjoberg, L. (2009) 'Introduction to Security Studies: Feminist Contributions' *Security Studies* 18, 2: 183–213.

Sow, Ndeye (2006) *Gender and Conflict Transformation in Great Lakes Region of Africa*. London: International Alert. www.glow-boell.de/media/de/txt_rubrik_2/Nde ye_Sow_FGmai06.pdf

Spiegel, P. B. (2004) 'HIV/AIDS among Conflict-affected and Displaced Populations: Dispelling Myths and Taking Action' *Disasters* 28, 3: 322–39.

Spiegel, P. B. and Nankoe, A (2004) 'UNHCR, HIV/AIDS and Refugees: Lessons Learned' *Forced Migration Review* 19: 21–23.

Spiegel, P. B., Bennedsen, A. R., Claass, J., Bruns, L., Patterson, N., Yiweza, D., and Schilperoord, M. (2007) 'Prevalence of HIV infection in conflict-affected and displaced people in seven sub-Saharan African countries: a systematic review', *Lancet* 360: 2187–95.

Steiner, B., Benner, M. T., Sondorp, E., Schmitz, K. P., Mesmer, U. and Rosenberger, S. (2009) Sexual Violence in the protracted conflict of DRC programming for rape survivors in south Kivu. *Conflict and Health* 3, 3.

Stern, M. (2006) '"We" the Subject: The power and Failure of (In) Security' *Security Dialogue* 37, 2: 187–205.

Szreter, S. and Fisher, K. (2010) *Sex Before the Sexual Revolution: Intimate Life in England 1918–1963*. Cambridge: Cambridge University Press.

Stone-Mediatore, S. (1998) 'Chnadra Mohanty and the Revaluing of "Experience"' *Hypatia* 13, 2: 116–33.

Susser, I. (2009) *AIDS, Sex and Culture: Global Politics and Survival in Southern Africa*. New York: Wiley-Blackwell

Tickner, A. (1997) 'You Just Don't Understand: Troubled Engagements Between Feminists and IR Theorists'. *International Studies Quarterly* 41: 611–32.

Tilly, C. (1999) *Durable Inequality.* Berkeley: University of California Press.

Tripodi, P. and Patel, P. (2002)'The Global Impact of HIV/AIDS on Peace support Operations' *International Peacekeeping* 9, 3: 51–66.

UN (2000) 'Resolution 1308 on the responsibility of the Security Council in the maintenance of international peace and security: HIV/AIDS and international peacekeeping operations-Adopted by the Security Council at its 4172nd meeting' 17 July 2000. S/RES/1308. http://daccessdds.un.org/doc/UNDOC/GEN/N00/536/02/PDF/N0053602.pdf?OpenElement

UNAIDS (2003) 'HIV/AIDS prevention and care among armed forces and UN peacekeepers: The case of Eritrea. In *Engaging Uniformed Services in the Fight Against AIDS.* Fighting AIDS Case Study 1. Geneva: UNAIDS.

——(2009) *Burundi Country Report.* Geneva: UNAIDS. www.unaids.org/en/regionsco untries/countries/burundi/

——(2010) *Burundi Country Progress Report.* http://data.unaids.org/pub/Report/2010/burundi_2010_country_progress_report_fr.pdf

UNDDR (2008) *Burundi.* United Nations Disarmament, Demobilization and Reintegration Resource Centre. www.unddr.org/countryprogrammes.php?c=17.

UNHCR (2010) *UNHCR Statistical Online Population Database: Sources, Methods and Data Considerations.* www.unhcr.org/45c06c662.html.

United States Institute of Peace (USIP) (2001) *Special Report: AIDS and Violent Conflict in Africa* Washington, DC: USIP.

Uvin, Peter (2009) *Life After Violence: A People's Story of Burundi.* London: Zed Books. www.unaids.org/documents/20101123_GlobalReport_Chap1_em.pdf.

van Wyk, B., Strebel, A., Peltzer, K., and Skinner, D. (2006) *Community-level behavioural interventions for HIV prevention in sub-Saharan Africa.* Cape Town: HSRC Press.

Vaughan, C. (2010) '"When the road is full of potholes, I wonder they are bringing condoms?" Social spaces for understanding young Papua New Guineans' health-related knowledge and health-promoting action' *AIDS Care* 22, 2: 1644–51.

Very, W. and Boshoff, H. (2006) *A Case Study for Burundi: Disarmament, Demobilization and Reintegration During the Transition in Burundi: A Technical Analysis.* Pretoria: ISS Publications. http://unddr.org/docs/DDR_during_the_transition.pdf.

Vielajus, M. and Haeringer, N. (2011) 'Transnational Networks of "Self-Realization": An Alternative Form of Struggle for Global Justice', in M. Albrow and H. Seckinelgin (eds) *Globality and the Absence of Justice: Global Civil Society 2011.* London: Palgrave.

Watkins, S. C. and Swidler, A. (2009) 'Hearsay ethnography: Conversational journals as a method for studying culture in action' *Poetics* Vol. 37: 162–84.

Watt, N. (2008) *Burundi: Biography of a Small African Country.* London: Hurst and Company.

WFN (2010) *BURUNDI 23 and 29 Jul 2010 African Former Hot Spot Elects Legislators.* www.newsahead.com/preview/2010/07/23/burundi-23-29-jul-2010-african-former-hot -spot-elects-legislators/index.php.

Whiteside, A., de Waal, A., and Gebre-Tensae, T. (2006) 'AIDS, Security and The Military in Africa: A Sober Appraisal', *African Affairs* 105, 419: 201–18.

WHO (2005) *Burundi.* Geneva: WHO. www.who.int/hiv/HIVCP_BDI.pdf.

Wibben, A. T. R. (2008) 'Human Security: Toward an Opening' *Security Dialogue* 39, 4: 455–62.

Willems, R., Kleingeld, J. and van Leeuwen, M. (2010) *Connecting Community Security and DDR Experiences from Burundi.* The Netherlands: PSD Network.

www.psdnetwork.nl/documenten/publications/20101101_Connecting_Community_S ecurity_and_DDR.pdf.

Wynne, B. (2002) 'Seasick on the Third Wave? Subverting the Hegemony of Propositionalism: response to Collins and Evans', *Social Studies of Science* 33, 3: 401–17.

Yeager, R., Hendrix, C. W., and Kingma, S. (2000), 'International military human immunodeficiency virus/acquired immunodeficiency syndrome policies and programs: strengths and limitations in current practice', *Military Medicine* 165, 2: 87–92.

Index

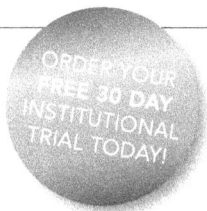

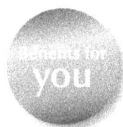

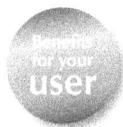

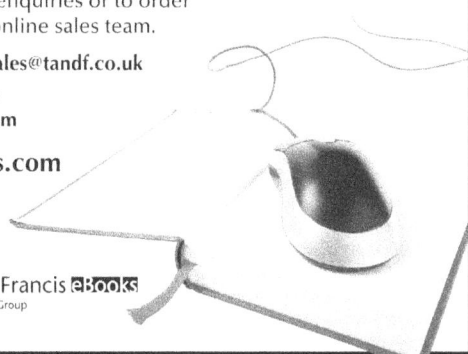

For Product Safety Concerns and Information please contact our EU
representative GPSR@taylorandfrancis.com
Taylor & Francis Verlag GmbH, Kaufingerstraße 24, 80331 München, Germany